soft lens fitting

For Elsevier:

Commissioning Editor: Robert Edwards
Development Editor: Kim Benson
Project Manager: Emma Riley
Design: George Ajayi
Illustrations Manager: Bruce Hogarth

eye essentials

soft lens fitting

Andrew Franklin BSc, FBCO, DOrth, DCLP
Professional Programme Tutor, Boots Opticians
Examiner, College of Optometrists, UK
Optometrist in private practice, Gloucestershire, UK

Ngaire Franklin BSc, FC Optom, DCLP
Examiner, College of Optometrists, UK
Optometrist in private practice, Herefordshire, UK

SERIES EDITORS

Sandip Doshi PhD, MCOptom
Optometrist in private practice, Hove, East Sussex, UK
Examiner, College of Optometrists, London, UK
Formerly Clinical Editor, Optician

William Harvey MCOptom
Visiting Clinician and Director of Visual Impairment Clinic, City University, London, UK
Professional Programme Tutor for Boots Opticians Ltd
Clinical Editor, Optician, Reed Business Information, Sutton, UK

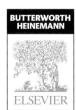

BUTTERWORTH
HEINEMANN

ELSEVIER

EDINBURGH LONDON NEW YORK OXFORD
PHILADELPHIA ST LOUIS SYDNEY TORONTO 2007

ELSEVIER
BUTTERWORTH
HEINEMANN

© 2007, Elsevier Limited. All rights reserved.
First published 2007

No part of this publication may be reproduced, stored in a retrieval system, or transmitted in any form or by any means, electronic, mechanical, photocopying, recording or otherwise, without the prior permission of the Publishers. Permissions may be sought directly from Elsevier's Health Sciences Rights Department, 1600 John F. Kennedy Boulevard, Suite 1800, Philadelphia, PA 19103-2899, USA: phone: (+1) 215 239 3804; fax: (+1) 215 239 3805; or, e-mail: *healthpermissions@elsevier.com*. You may also complete your request on-line via the Elsevier homepage (http: www.elsevier.com), by selecting 'Support and contact' and then 'Copyright and Permission'.

ISBN-13: 978-0-7506-8856-7
ISBN-10: 0-7506-8856-4

British Library Cataloguing in Publication Data
A catalogue record for this book is available from the British Library.

Library of Congress Cataloging in Publication Data
A catalog record for this book is available from the Library of Congress.

Note
Knowledge and best practice in this field are constantly changing. As new research and experience broaden our knowledge, changes in practice, treatment and drug therapy may become necessary or appropriate. Readers are advised to check the most current information provided (i) on procedures featured or (ii) by the manufacturer of each product to be administered, to verify the recommended dose or formula, the method and duration of administration, and contraindications. It is the responsibility of the practitioner, relying on their own experience and knowledge of the patient, to make diagnoses, to determine dosages and the best treatment for each individual patient, and to take all appropriate safety precautions. To the fullest extent of the law, neither the publisher nor the editors assumes any liability for any injury and/or damage.

The Publisher

Printed in Europe

Contents

Foreword vii
Introduction ix
Dedication xi
Acknowledgments xiii

1. Initial consultation   **1**

2. Soft lens materials   **25**

3. Spherical lens fitting   **35**

4. Soft lenses for astigmatism   **57**

5. Soft contact lenses in presbyopia   **69**

6. Extended wear and silicone hydrogels   **83**

7. Collection and lens care   **101**

8. Aftercare   **123**

9. Complications and management   **135**

10. Tinted and therapeutic lenses   **161**

Index   171

Foreword

Eye Essentials is a series of books intended to cover the core skills required by the eye care practitioner in general and/or specialized practice. It consists of books covering a wide range of topics ranging from: routine eye examination to assessment and management of low vision; assessment and investigative techniques to digital imaging; case reports and law to contact lenses.

Authors known for their interest and expertise in their particular subject have contributed books to this series. The reader will know many of them, as they have published widely within their respective fields. Each author has addressed key topics in their subject in a practical rather than theoretical approach, hence each book has a particular relevance to everyday practice.

Each book in the series follows a similar format and has been designed to allow the reader to ascertain information easily and quickly. Each chapter has been produced in a user-friendly format, thus providing the reader with a rapid-reference book that is easy to use in the consulting room or in the practitioner's free time.

Optometry and dispensing optics are continually developing professions, with the emphasis in each being redefined as we learn more from research and as technology stamps its mark. The *Eye Essentials* series is particularly relevant to the practitioner's requirements and as such will appeal to students, graduates sitting professional examinations and qualified practitioners alike. We hope you enjoy reading these books as much as we have enjoyed producing them.

Sandip Doshi
Bill Harvey

Introduction

Towards the end of a sight test, one of those utterances that the busy practitioner may dread is 'I was wondering whether to go for contact lenses'. Practitioners who do not regularly fit contact lenses are often convinced that it has all become a bit too complicated, and that contact lenses are best left to the experts, whoever they are. Patients are discouraged from too active an interest by rather vaguely negative advice. Of course, there are practitioners who actively encourage their patients to use contact lenses, but in the UK they are a small minority. Part of the reason may be that Britons are uncomfortable with the active promotion of anything, for fear of being thought of as 'pushy' or (brace yourselves) 'showing off'. However, this seems a poor explanation for a UK contact lens market of 7% of the population, compared with a US market of 15%. There may also be a confidence factor at work here. Many UK practitioners have lost touch with modern contact lens practice, or at least aspects of it. The reasons vary. Some small rural practices may simply not generate very much contact lens work at all, or little beyond the odd daily disposable. Some busy practices employ contact lens fitters, and the optometrists rarely see the contact lens patients except for their spectacle refractions. Some optometrists have taken a career break, to raise children or pursue a different career path. After a few years in full-time management of either type, the contact lens world can appear dauntingly unfamiliar. When the authors began fitting lenses, there were only a few soft lenses available, so lens material selection was easy. Some of them wetted better than others, but none of them transmitted a decent amount of oxygen. In those simpler times, aftercare was also relatively easy. The slit-lamps that we had were not good enough to see much (indeed, it was not uncommon to practise without one), and when we did see something, we either did not know what caused it or did not have lenses that would deal with it. As with certain soap operas, you could take a year off them and not have a lot to catch up with. These days we can see more and do more, and have a huge and bewildering choice of options. What is even worse, so do the patients. At one time, professional knowledge could be jealously hoarded, but now anyone with a computer and half an hour can gain access to astonishing levels of technical and clinical information. This has spawned that most dreaded of patients – the 'Internet Bully'. Usually male, and not promoted to the levels that his intellect demands (at least in his opinion), the Internet Bully surfs the web for ammunition with which to harass his optometrist. (And probably his doctor, dentist, and any other sort of 'ist' he consults.)

This book and its companion volume (*Rigid Gas-Permeable Lenses*) are aimed at those colleagues who wish to re-enter the contact lens mainstream, as well as those entering it for the first time as students and pre-registered optometrists. It also aims to meet the requirements suggested in our new General Optical Council entry level competencies, to which all qualified practitioners are meant to adhere if they are to maintain their place on the General Optical Council register. It is not intended to be comprehensive or overly academic, but should enable the practitioner to give sound advice to their patients, and should provide a basis on which to build should they wish to specialize further. And you should be able to handle the Internet Bully too.

Dedication

Such is the pace of change, most contact lens books go out of date rapidly. So read it fast!

Acknowledgments

We are grateful to Chanel King and Heidi Harvey for their assistance with photographs.

1
Initial consultation

Introduction   2
Should this patient be wearing contact lenses?   2
Ocular health   3
General health   3
Visual factors   4
Psychological factors   5
Occupation and lifestyle   6
Financial considerations   6
Soft or rigid?   7
Patient examination   8
General observation of the eye and adnexa   8
Assessment of the palpebral conjunctiva   9
Assessment of the bulbar conjunctiva   11
The tear film   12
General examination of the cornea   15
Specific examination of the cornea   19
Blue light examination of the cornea   22
References   24

Introduction

The initial consultation with a prospective contact lens wearer is an important dialogue between the practitioner and patient that has a number of goals:

1. to establish whether the patient is suitable for any type of contact lens correction
2. to identify the optimal contact lens correction for the individual patient
3. to establish reasonable expectations for the performance of the lenses and care system
4. to educate the patient so that their use of the lenses will be safe and sensible
5. to determine baseline information that can be used to monitor change that can influence future management decisions.

The majority of contact lens fitting is elective (i.e. non-therapeutic), and the patient will exert a degree of control over the lenses selected and their compliance with care systems. The principle of informed choice is important here. The patient must be given enough information to make appropriate decisions (i.e. those the practitioner approves of). The days when the practitioner held a monopoly on information have long departed. Most patients who present for contact lens fitting will also possess a computer and internet access. Therefore, information that is incorrect or out of date will be easily detected, with consequent loss of credibility for the practitioner. It is important that practitioners keep themselves well informed on current developments.

Should this patient be wearing contact lenses?

There are few absolute contraindications to contact lens wear these days, although there are many more issues that may limit it, or make it more complicated for the patient or practitioner.

Ophthalmologic consultation is essential before fitting any eye with active corneal pathology, and infective conditions should be eliminated before fitting to minimize the risk of microbial keratitis. The patient should be aware of any factors that will increase their risk, so that they can weigh this against the benefits.

Ocular health

1. Ocular surface disorders may cause problems:
   (a) Recurrent erosions may be associated with anomalies of the basement membrane of the epithelium. In severe cases, a bandage lens may be indicated.
   (b) Recurrent bacterial infections will increase the risk of microbial keratitis significantly and in general contact lenses should be avoided in such patients.
2. Dry eye is the most commonly encountered complication. The effect on contact lens wear can be predicted by the severity of symptoms and corneal staining encountered before fitting. People with milder symptoms can usually be given contact lenses, at least for part-time wear.
3. Meibomian gland dysfunction (MGD) can be a significant factor in contact lens intolerance and its prevalence is age-related. Fewer than 20% of patients under 20 years of age present with it, but two-thirds of over-65s are found to have MGD.

General health

Both systemic pathology and the medication used to treat it may be significant factors when considering contact lenses.

1. Allergies may be associated with a poor tear film and a tendency to develop inflammatory reactions to solutions or lens deposits. Daily disposable lenses or non-preserved solutions may be indicated.
2. Chronic infections such as sinusitis or catarrh may cause excessive mucus in the tears. The eyes may also be more prone to infection.

3. **Hypertensive** patients are prone to dry eye because of the β-blockers or diuretics used to treat their condition. A number of other medications have similar effects on the tear film. Common examples include antibiotics, antihistamines and psychomimetics such as diazepam, amitriptyline, chlordiazepoxide and thioridazine.

4. **Thyroid dysfunction** tends to cause both dry eye and poor blinking.

5. **Hormonal changes** associated with pregnancy, lactation and the menopause may be associated with a tendency for corneal edema and mucus accumulation. Generally, it is unwise to commence fitting during pregnancy. The tear film may also be affected, and traditionally the use of oral contraceptives has also been assumed to have similar effects. However, a recent study (Tomlinson et al, 2001) did not support this assumption, possibly because modern contraceptive pills contain lower doses of hormone.

6. **Diabetic** patients may have a slightly higher oxygen requirement to avoid edema and an unstable refractive error. The cornea may be a little more fragile, and wound healing takes a little longer. However, a study by O'Donnell et al (2001) found that, provided that the diabetes was well controlled, no extra risk was associated with daily wear. For extended wear, the reduced handling of lenses during insertion and removal might favor a fragile cornea, but there are insufficient data on complications with this modality, mainly because few practitioners are keen on anything beyond part-time wear. Daily disposable lenses are popular, but silicone hydrogel lenses may give the best physiologic response, due to their greater oxygen transmission.

Visual factors

Several issues may be revealed by the patient's history:

1. Myopes will have a larger retinal image with contact lenses. This may improve Snellen acuity, although it will reduce the field of vision a little.

2. Myopes who wear their spectacles for reading may find that they miss the base-in prism induced when they look through the near centers. The result can be a decompensated exophoria. Those who habitually read without spectacles will find that they have to accommodate more when wearing spectacles. Those on the edges of presbyopia may struggle. Furthermore, the extra accommodation required will also cause extra convergence, which will tend to make the patient relatively esophoric.

3. Hyperopes will have a smaller retinal image with contact lenses. This improves their field of vision but may reduce their visual acuity. Many hyperopes only wear their spectacles for near-vision tasks, and correction of their refractive error for distance may induce exophoria. However, hyperopic early presbyopes may find that contact lenses, particularly aspheric ones, help them to read.

4. Prismatic correction is impractical in contact lenses, unless it is vertical. To correct this, overall prism ballast can be used. It is theoretically possible to prescribe horizontal prism in a rigid gas permeable (RGP) lens by incorporating platinum ballast, but it has rarely been done and even less often been successful.

Psychological factors

The psychological traits of the patient may well influence their ability to adapt to contact lenses, and to look after them. A certain amount of intelligence is required to cope with lens care, preferably linked with a modicum of common sense. Extroverts may well adapt easily, but can also become a little creative with their lens care, since they tend to guess if unsure. Introverts may be detail-obsessed and may find adaptation a challenge, particularly if they require exacting standards of vision.

Most elective fitting is driven by vanity, and the patient who is prepared to admit this will probably be honest about compliance after fitting. Some patients will invent spurious reasons for wanting lenses. The patient whose stated motivation involves the avoidance of fogging spectacle lenses may be just as evasive at their aftercare visits.

The perceived improvement in appearance that contact lenses may bring is a powerful motivation in many patients, particularly in those with high spectacle prescriptions. It may be even greater in those with iris anomalies, corneal scars or inoperable squints. It is often observed that such patients become more outgoing and optimistic when they wear contact lenses. However, there are some patients who expect contact lenses to change an unhappy life, and they must be approached with caution. In all cases, the patient must have realistic expectations of what can be achieved. In general, a slight overstating of the difficulties likely to be encountered can be helpful. If the patient is anticipating some complications while you optimize the fit, they will not become anxious. If you sort things out in less time, the patient may think you are a genius.

It is worth bearing in mind that patients attending for sight tests have been found to have higher stress levels than those visiting the dentist. Contact lens patients have more reason than most to be nervous, so attention to phraseology and body language is important. Light-colored clothing may make the practitioner less threatening, and an informal manner also helps.

Occupation and lifestyle

Some environments are unsuitable or challenging for contact lenses, because of contamination or extremes of temperature. There are also certain occupations in which contact lens wear is discouraged, sometimes on rather dubious grounds. Hygiene is always an important consideration, and a certain amount of lens handling is involved, during which rough or calloused hands may present a challenge to the lenses.

Financial considerations

There is a tendency to overemphasize this aspect, and practitioners sometimes offer lenses that are less than optimal, on grounds of cost. Realistically, the average contact lens wearer probably spends more on a pair of shoes, and probably has more than one pair. Patients should be offered the best lens for their visual and physiologic needs, and any compromise on financial grounds should be understood properly by the patient. Furthermore, a desire to save money on the lenses may also have implications for compliance with lens care.

Soft or rigid?

When the authors started fitting contact lenses, this was a question that required some thought. Rigid lenses were more commonly fitted, as the soft lenses of the day were not particularly good. These days, however, soft lenses are the preferred option in most cases. There are lenses to fit nearly every patient, and workable toric, multifocal and colored lenses are easily available. With the advent of silicone hydrogel lenses, oxygen is rarely an issue, and even extended wear is a practical proposition. Daily disposables even circumvent the chore of cleaning and storing the lenses. The biggest advantage of soft lenses, however, is that they are comfortable from the outset, unlike rigid lenses, which require adaptation before acceptable levels of comfort are attained. In this world of instant gratification, people are rarely prepared to invest the time and effort to adapt to RGP lenses, but there are still some patients for whom this type of lens should be the first choice:

1. Patients with irregular astigmatism due to corneal damage or keratoconus will only obtain satisfactory vision with RGP lenses.
2. Existing rigid lens wearers may not be satisfied with the visual performance of soft lenses.
3. Patients with particularly exacting visual requirements will probably see better with RGP lenses. This is particularly true for presbyopes.
4. High-minus prescriptions will result in lenses that are thickest at the edge of the optic zone. On a hydrogel lens, oxygen transmission is likely to be poor. It will be better on a silicone

hydrogel lens, but an RGP lens will give a much better oxygen level around the limbal area.

5. Patients who have limbal neovascularization from previous soft lens wear will be better off with RGP lenses, although silicone hydrogel lenses may be an option.

Patient examination

The examination of the patient can begin as naked-eye observation during the initial dialogue. In particular, at this stage, do the following:

1. Make a note of the patient's **complexion**. Patients with auburn hair and freckles tend to have more sensitive corneas.
2. Note **eye color**. Blue-eyed patients tend to be more sensitive, especially with rigid lenses.
3. **Lid position** will be important, particularly with RGP, toric and multifocal lenses. If the lid position is unusual, a diagram should be drawn illustrating it.

The rest of the examination is conducted with the major slit-lamp. The examination has three phases:

1. general observation of the eye and adnexa
2. general observation of the cornea with white light and medium magnification
3. specific examination of the cornea with white and cobalt blue light.

General observation of the eye and adnexa

General observation of the eye and adnexa with a low-magnification setting may be conducted with focal illumination and a wide beam, but often a far better view can be obtained by the use of diffuse illumination. The diffuser gives the effect of a much larger light source, and gives the eye a more natural appearance, as well as allowing more of the eye to be illuminated at one time. Shadows tend to be minimized, allowing detail to be seen. On the other hand, some loss of information on texture and topographic variation may occur, as the shadows provided by tangential focal illumination may highlight this. A combination of the two forms of illumination is required.

With diffuse illumination, and low magnification, attention is spread widely, encompassing the whole field of vision. This is ideal for a general survey of the area. As the beam width narrows, and the magnification rises, greater detail can be seen, but of a correspondingly more limited area. If we only performed the high-magnification examination, we would probably miss something significant while our attention was focused on some tiny detail elsewhere. We should therefore look at the eye in the same way as we would look for a set of keys, with a general reconnaissance of every room before we demolish the sofa.

The following areas should be covered:

1. The external aspects of the lids, looking for signs of inflammation and swelling.
2. The lashes should be observed for signs of:
   (a) **ectropion,** which may be associated with poor drainage
   (b) **entropion** and **trichiasis**.
3. The lid margins, looking for signs of **blepharitis,** which can be associated with changes in both conjunctiva and cornea, and may cause an unstable tear film that could affect contact lens wear. Chronic blepharitis may be encountered as the anterior form, either staphylococcal or sebhorrhoeic. There is also a posterior type (MGD).

Assessment of the palpebral conjunctiva

To examine the conjunctiva, broad-beam diffuse illumination is used initially, with the emphasis on assessing the degree, depth and location of hyperemia. This may then be followed by more detailed examinations using focal illumination. Dyes and stains, and filters, may be used to reveal areas of damage.

Severity may be indicated using a grading scale. There are several published grading systems, but correlation between them

Table 1.1 **Grading scale for assessment of the palpebral conjunctiva**

Lens type	Appearance	Significance
0	Normal	None
1	Slight	Note but no action
2	Moderate	May require action
3	Severe	Requires action
4	Very severe	Refer for medical intervention

is a little hit and miss, and none is accepted universally. The authors tend to favor a simple intuitive scale for all observations, as it saves time in trying to fit the observation to the photographs or diagrams used in the published versions. If I were a patient, I am not sure that I would be very impressed if my practitioner was constantly referring to charts. The intuitive scale used is similar to the one described by Woods (Table 1.1).

If the observations do not quite fit the gradings, we can use plus and minus increments to convert the scale into a nine-point one, which should be sensitive enough for even the most pedantic observer.

The **distribution of hyperemia** is best recorded as a diagram. Distribution is important. A discrete leash of dilated blood vessels on the bulbar conjunctiva may point to a phlycten. Interpalpebral redness may be associated with drying or with a hypersensitivity reaction to an airborne irritant. Where the hyperemia is greater under one or both lids, we may be dealing with 'innocent bystander' (secondary hypersensitivity) reactions resulting from an inflamed palpebral conjunctiva.

The **depth of hyperemia** is important in differentiating mere conjunctivitis from episcleritis, scleritis and uveitis, and grading is useful. The injection associated with conjunctivitis tends to be bright red and greatest towards the fornices. Going deeper, the hyperemia associated with episcleritis tends to be salmon-pink, and wedge-shaped, with the apex towards the limbus due to the radial arrangement of the vessels, although the 20% who have the nodular form will show a more circumscribed area of redness. Scleritis produces a purplish hue that is diffuse and present all the way to the fornices. Uveitis itself produces deep injection that is most intense around the limbus.

Assessment of the bulbar conjunctiva

In general, the examination of the bulbar conjunctiva will proceed in three sweeps, taking in the upper, middle and lower thirds, with the lids pulled back to see what lies below. In order to view the palpebral conjunctiva, the lids must be everted. Professional Qualifying Examination (PQE) candidates invariably seem to use cotton buds for this purpose, but with practice in many patients the lids can be everted using the fingers alone, and the ubiquitous cotton bud is not an ideal tool for the purpose anyway. The end tends to be too bulbous, and teasing out the fibers will often result in a more useful implement, being easier to insert behind the tarsal margin. The following should be noted:

1. The pattern of any hyperemia, particularly if contact lens-related papillary conjunctivitis (CLPC) is suspected, as it tends to favor the upper lid.
2. Internal hordeola and concretions, which appear as discrete yellowish dots. These are of little significance unless they break through to the surface, in which case they are easily removed medically, using a needle.
3. Follicles and papillae with diffuse white light initially to look for hyperemia, but focal illumination, directed tangentially, is useful to show the texture, as the shadows will be more obvious. With fluorescein installed, surface texture is enhanced, as the dye collects in the channels between the swellings (Fig. 1.1).
   (a) **Follicles** are lymphatic in origin, so they are avascular. They appear as multiple, discrete, slightly elevated bodies that are translucent and shaped rather like rice grains (arborio rather than basmati). As they grow, they displace the conjunctival vessels, so they can appear with a vascular

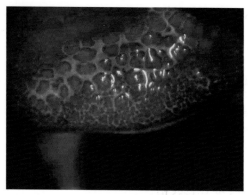

Figure 1.1 Fluorescein emphasizes elevations on the palpebral surface

capsule surrounding the base. They are generally small, but can measure up to 5 mm in severe or unusually prolonged disease.

(b) **Papillae** have their origin in the palpebral conjunctival tissue, and consist of a central vascular tuft surrounded by a diffuse infiltrate, largely composed of white blood cells. They can only occur where the conjunctival epithelium is attached to the underlying levels by fibrous septa. This restricts them to the palpebral conjunctiva and limbal area. Giant papillae occur when these septa are ruptured.

The tear film

A series of observations can be made on the tear film:

1. **Tear prism height** may be seen by observing the tear prism in section. The normal tear prism is about 0.2–0.4 mm in height, and appears convex in section. A scanty tear film will have a low meniscus (less than 0.2 mm), which will appear concave. Irregularity of the prism along the lid edge suggests a poor tear film.

2. **Dust particles** and **bubbles** can be observed within the lower rivus under high magnification. In the normal tear film, particles on the surface move more slowly than deeper ones, due to surface tension. If the speed of particles is too high, a thin, watery tear film is indicated. Immobile particles reveal excessive viscosity in the tear film.

3. The **tear break-up time** (TBUT) may be assessed by instilling fluorescein, and then waiting for a few seconds for the tear film to stabilize while the patient blinks. The eye is illuminated with a broad beam with the cobalt filter. The patient is then instructed not to blink, and the time noted for dark spots or streaks to appear in the tear layer as it breaks up. Normally, this would take 15–20 seconds, and anything below 10 seconds is probably abnormal. Where the same area consistently breaks up rapidly, this is due to a surface irregularity rather than dry eye.

4. **Non-invasive tear break-up time** (NIBUT) can be measured by observing keratometer mires, or a Keeler Tearscope-Plus may be used to project a grid pattern onto the eye's surface, which is then observed for distortion as the tear film breaks. Typical NIBUT times for normal subjects are about 40 seconds with this method.

5. The **Tearscope** can also be used to observe interference patterns in the tear film, allowing an estimate of the tear thickness to be made. If a Tearscope is not available, some idea of the quality of the tears may be obtained if the first Purkinje image of the slit beam is observed, especially if the illumination is reduced and the beam narrowed. Colored fringes around the Purkinje image, seen in conjunction with an irregular tear prism, strongly suggest a poor tear film (Fig. 1.2).

6. **Mucous strands** and **debris** in the tears can be an early sign of dry eye. This occurs as the mucin layer becomes contaminated with lipid as the tear film breaks up. Mucin may also combine with cellular debris in more severe cases and form filaments, which are attached to the epithelial surface and move with each blink. Mucous plaques, whitish-gray translucent lesions of varying shape, may appear in concert with the filaments. Fluorescein will reveal punctate

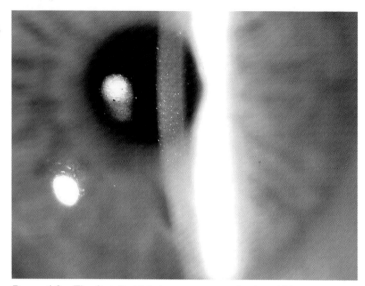

Figure 1.2 The first Purkinje image may reveal colored fringes indicative of an unstable lipid layer

epitheliopathy, either in the inferior portion of the cornea or in the interpalpebral area.

7. Damage may also be revealed by the use of **rose bengal** stain. This stains dead and devitalized cells and mucus red. Typically, dry-eye patients show staining of the interpalpebral bulbar conjunctiva, with two triangular areas of stain either side of the cornea, with their apices towards the inner and outer canthi. Mucous strands, filaments and plaques will also show up better with rose bengal. The drawback to rose bengal is that it is a considerable ocular irritant, and, as luck would have it, this quality is rather worse in dry-eye patients. **Lissamine green SF** (wool green, light green SF), which stains dead cells and mucus blue–green, and is less of an irritant, appeared in the 1960s as an alternative to rose bengal. It is available in the USA as impregnated strips, but is at present unavailable commercially in the UK.

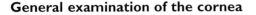
General examination of the cornea

The magnification used for the initial examination of the cornea is important. If this is set low, the whole cornea (indeed, half of the patient's face) can be covered in one fell sweep. Unfortunately, very little of clinical significance can be detected. This may be initially reassuring for both patient and practitioner, but the longer-term consequences for both are unattractive. An initial examination at too high a magnification would take a rather long time, even assuming that the full consciousness of both parties can be maintained for the duration. It is also far too easy to become lost if the field of vision is too small to contain reference points to navigate by. Therefore, initially, the cornea is examined with medium magnification, set so that the whole cornea may be seen in three horizontal sweeps. If an anomaly is detected, the magnification can be increased to allow a closer look.

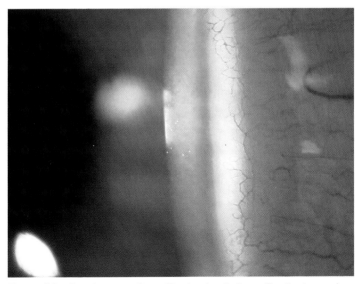

Figure 1.3 Simultaneous direct illumination, indirect illumination and retroillumination

This angle between the slit beam and the visual axis of the microscope is important for a number of reasons. It allows deeper structures to be observed without an overlay of reflected light from more superficial structures, and this enhances clarity considerably. The wider the slit beam, the greater becomes the angle between the beam and the microscope required to achieve this separation. Another happy consequence of an angled beam is that it is possible to view the cornea by direct illumination, indirect illumination and retroillumination simultaneously (Fig. 1.3).

The area of cornea where the beam strikes is directly illuminated, and, if the observer looks to either side of this bright area, the cornea may be seen in indirect illumination. Opacities will scatter light and be seen as light areas against a dark background (Fig. 1.4). A dark background is essential for this, so the room lighting should be off.

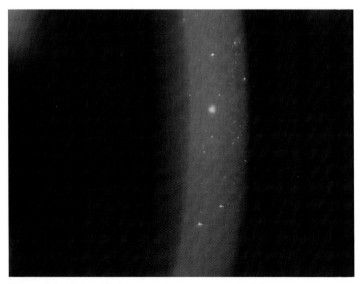

Figure 1.4 Direct illumination shows opacities as light areas

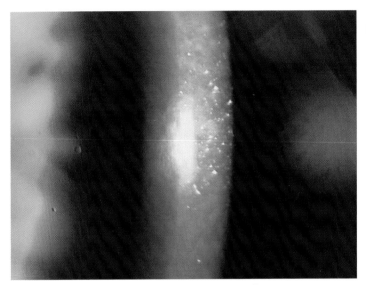

Figure 1.5 Retroillumination shows opacities in silhouette

To the opposite side from that from which the beam is directed will be an area of cornea that is backlit by reflected light from the iris. Opacities here will appear in silhouette, dark against a light background (Fig. 1.5).

For the initial examination of the cornea, the beam width should be set at about 2 mm or so, which will illuminate a thick slice of the cornea termed a **parallelepiped**. An angle of 45–60° between beam and microscope allows some appreciation of depth, since the edge of the parallelepiped on the opposite side to that from which the light is coming is, in effect, an optical section of sorts (Fig. 1.6).

The beam is slowly swept from the limbus to the central cornea. Most authorities recommend that the illumination is from the same side as the hemicornea being examined; that is, when the cornea to the left of the midline is being observed, the lamp is positioned to the left of the microscope, and the illumination system is swung round to the other side as the midline is

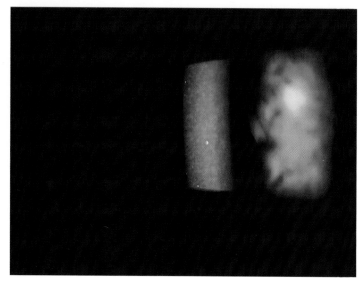

Figure 1.6   A parallelepiped

crossed. However, the authors prefer to sweep from limbus to limbus, with the illumination from each side in turn. Light bounced from the iris can then be employed to retroilluminate the limbal arcades on the 'wrong side'.

When the beam is directed to the limbus, it may be worth widening the beam momentarily and observing the cornea with the naked eye, particularly if the patient already wears polymethyl methacrylate (PMMA) or low-Dk RGP lenses (for an explanation of Dk, see Chapter 2). The light under these circumstances is internally reflected within the cornea, and a bright glow may be seen around the limbus. Dense central edema will cause the internally reflected light to scatter and produce a gray glow that can be seen against the dark pupil area. It is possible to decouple the instrument in order to view the cornea through the microscope, but it is rarely necessary since the demise of PMMA lenses. The technique is referred to as

sclerotic scatter, and it is really only a version of indirect illumination. Sclerotic scatter can also be useful when observing the limbal arcades. A 1–2 mm angled beam is directed at the sclera immediately adjacent to the limbus. The microscope remains coupled, but the attention is directed to the limbus and the area of the cornea immediately inside it. The limbal arcades can be seen, illuminated partly by internally reflected light and partly by light reflected back off the iris.

The sweeps are performed with the patient looking slightly down, level and slightly up, and new users should be careful to remember all three. For some reason, optometry students have the unfortunate habit of forgetting to look at the upper cornea, particularly if they look at the other parts first and detect any anomalies. The area of cornea under the lid is particularly likely to develop anomalies due to hypoxia, since oxygen levels are generally lower under the lid, and may also show 'innocent bystander' effects such as the keratitis associated with CLPC, due to close proximity to the lid. For this reason, it is a good idea to get into the habit of viewing the upper cornea first every time. At this stage, we are essentially looking for opacities:

1. Infiltrates indicate active or recently active inflammation. Some patients show one or more small, discrete infiltrates distributed at random. These are rarely significant, and are probably related to environmental pollution, but are worth noting, if only to avoid wasting time on them later.
2. Scars indicate past inflammation that may be related to infection.

Specific examination of the cornea

Examination at high magnification may be undertaken either because general examination has detected an anomaly, or because the history or symptoms of the patient suggest that a specific anomaly may be present. For example, an existing soft contact lens wearer might have microcysts or neovascularization. However, even patients with no history of contact lens wear may have microcysts or vacuoles, and it is important to note their presence in order to differentiate them from those caused by lenses.

Any anomaly of the cornea should be recorded in detail:

1. **Where is it?** Accurate recording of the distance from the limbus (or center) and the clock position makes it easier to find the anomaly again. The estimation of distances when the eye is under magnification is a challenge to the inexperienced microscopist, and this can cause unnecessary alarm in cases of suspected neovascularization, for example. Some slit-lamp microscopes have a graticule eyepiece, which can be useful when making quantitative observations. However, some observers (including the authors) find the graticule distracting. Reasonable estimates of dimensions may be made with a little practice by comparing the size of the object of attention with a known dimension. The visible diameter of the cornea is 11–12 mm, and the amount by which a normal soft lens exceeds it is about a millimeter all round. Alternatively, one can always hold a millimeter rule close to the anomaly (but be careful!).

2. **How big** and **how many?** With a wide beam and lowish magnification, the size of a large opacity, or the number of a multiple one, may be determined. Large single opacities may be associated with bacterial infection, or the later stages of herpetic ulceration, whereas multiple smaller ones may be caused by a non-microbial agent, or by a viral or protozoan infection.

3. **Color** and **density** are best assessed with direct illumination. Although most corneal lesions tend to be monochrome, a hemorrhage within the cornea would give rise to a red lesion, and a rust stain might betray a ferrous foreign body. Some of the less dense lesions are more or less invisible under direct illumination and may only appear under indirect illumination or retroillumination, the classic example being ghost vessels (see below). Oscillation of the beam so that the type of illumination alternates may be useful, and can be achieved either by use of

the joystick or by decoupling the instrument and swinging the illumination system independently.

4. The **depth** of an infiltrate or scar tends to correlate with the seriousness of its cause. Intraepithelial infiltrates are usually a response to a non-microbial trigger, although this may include bacterial exotoxins. The deeper, subepithelial and stromal infiltrates are more likely to be associated with infection, and may lead to scarring. Depth perception through a biomicroscope is a result of a composite impression from a series of observations and improves with practice. Experienced microscopists often appear to fidget with both the illuminator and the microscope, seemingly at random to the casual observer. However, valuable information can be gleaned from these maneuvers, even though much of it may be subliminal to the microscopist.

(a) Varying the position of the light source will affect the degree to which the scattered light from layers near to the surface will interfere with the clear resolution of objects in the deeper layers. Parallax between the object and the leading edge of the parallelepiped is also induced.

(b) Swinging the microscope will also create parallax between structures at different levels (see below).

(c) The microscope allows binocular fixation, so stereopsis may be used, provided that the array is sufficiently detailed.

(d) Not all layers of the cornea will be in focus at the same time, particularly at high magnification, when the depth of focus is small.

(e) By far the best way to determine the depth of a lesion within the cornea is to narrow the beam, and observe the resultant thin optical section through a microscope set at a considerable angle to the illuminating system.

(f) The other very useful property of a thin section is that elevations and depressions in an interface or surface will cause the beam to deviate. Elevations move the beam towards the side that the light beam is coming from; depressions bend it away from the source. Where the cornea is perforated, there will be a gap in the corneal section. To make the most of this effect, an angled beam is essential.

Blue light examination of the cornea

The use of fluorescein to examine epithelial integrity is a vital part of every corneal examination, and there is no valid reason not to do it. If there are concerns that a patient's soft lenses will be discolored, the patient can always be given a daily lens to wear home. Fluorescein colors the tear film rather than staining the tissue. Normally, the lipid membranes of the epithelial cells prevent ingress of the substance, but if these are breached by trauma or disease, the tear layer gains access to deeper layers. The absorption spectrum and the degree of fluorescence depend on the pH peaking at 8. The underlying tissues, because they have a different pH to the surface, will fluoresce more, so the defect is shown up as a green area. In the deeper layers, the fluorescein does diffuse sideways, tending to exaggerate the area of the lesion, and this spread of fluorescein in the stroma may be a useful clue in itself when evaluating epithelial defects. When using the cobalt filter, it should be remembered that considerable light has been filtered out, and the rheostat adjusted to give a bright beam. Contrast may be considerably enhanced by the use of a yellow filter (Wratten no. 12 or no. 15) to eliminate blue light reflected from the cornea (Figure 1.7), although recently a lemon yellow filter has been found to be even more effective.

The magnification should also be appropriate. Fine punctate staining cannot be detected at low magnification and may be significant. Fluorescein in the tear film may make corneal staining more difficult to see. It helps if the instillation is frugal, as fluorescein will dye the patient's face or clothing at least as well as their corneas. A short delay (a minute or two) between instillation and observation is useful, to allow the tears to dilute the fluorescein. Fluorescein staining is best recorded as a diagram to illustrate its distribution, along with grading to indicate severity.

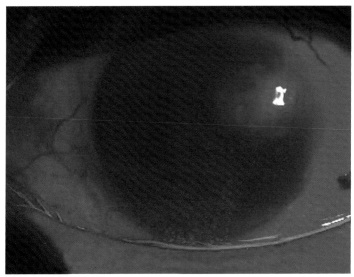

a

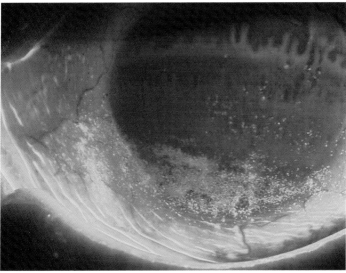

b

Figure 1.7 The absorption of blue reflected light (a) with a yellow filter (b) (courtesy of Topcon)

References

O'Donnell C, Efron N and Boulton AJM (2001) A prospective study of contact lens wear in diabetes mellitus. *Ophthalmic Physiol Optics* **21**: 127–138.

Tomlinson A, Pearce EI, Simmons PA and Blades K (2001) Effects of oral contraceptives on tear physiology. *Ophthalmic Physiol Optics* **21**: 9–16.

Woods R (1989) Quantitative slit lamp observations in contact lens practice. *J Brit Contact Lens Assoc.*, Scientific Meetings: 42–45.

2
Soft lens materials

Introduction   26
Classification of soft lens materials   28
Factors influencing water content   29
   The effects of decreased water content   30
   Silicone hydrogel   32
Reference   34
Further reading   34

Introduction

Soft contact lenses consist of two or more monomers polymerized together to form a copolymer. Copolymers are often referred to simply as 'polymers'. The concept of the 'washing line' is sometimes used to understand soft lens polymers. The washing line itself is a long polymer chain from which many hydrophilic groups (the 'wash') are suspended. At intervals, the washing lines are fastened to each other by cross-linkages. Cross-linkages stop the material falling apart.

The first soft contact lens material to appear was hydroxyethylmethacrylate, universally known as HEMA. (Strictly speaking, HEMA is the monomer form, and the correct term for the polymer is polyHEMA.) HEMA has a free hydroxyl group that can bind with water, which renders it hydrophilic. HEMA in its dry form is hard and glassy. As it hydrates, or 'plasticizes', spaces within the lens (the pores) enlarge and fill with water, giving the lens a rather sponge-like structure. Higher-water-content lenses usually have larger pores. HEMA is a comfortable material to wear but it is fragile, and easy to soil and discolor, and bacteria find it fairly easy to adhere to. Furthermore, its water content is 38% and its Dk is approximately 9, which is rather too low to maintain corneal health even for daily wear. For hydrogel materials, Dk and water content have a linear relationship (Fig. 2.1).

The actual oxygen transmission depends on the thickness of the lens, but there are practical limits on how thin the lens can be before its fragility becomes intolerable.

In order to improve Dk, the water content must be increased and other monomers must be added. Most lenses today still contain some HEMA, along with one or more extra ingredients.

1. Methacrylic acid (MA) adds an extra hydroxyl group to the polymer, which increases the water content. It is often used in rigid gas permeable (RGP) materials to improve wetting. It is

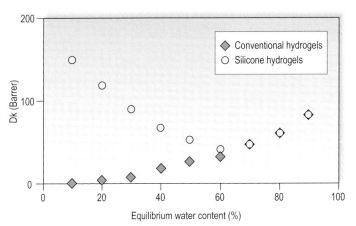

Figure 2.1 Linear relationship between Dk and water content (reproduced with permission from Efron Contact Lens Practice, Butterworth-Heinemann, 2002)

found in the familiar Acuvue (Johnson and Johnson) lenses as well as in a number of 55% monthly replacement lenses.
2. Agrylamide contains a carboxyl group that attracts water. It is found in Hydrocurve (Wesley-Jessen) lenses.
3. *N*-vinyl pyrrolidone (NVP or VP) also has a carboxyl group. It can be used with HEMA or without it.

Other common ingredients found include methyl methacrylate (MMA), which makes the lens stronger and more rigid, and ethylene glycol dimethacrylate, which is a cross-linking agent.

NVP and MMA are the basis of some Bausch and Lomb lenses (e.g. Medallist). Glycerylmethyl methacrylate (GMA) has been used by Wesley-Jessen in combination with MMA. The glyceryl supplies the hydrophilic element, and the MMA provides better optical performance than is found in HEMA lenses. The drawbacks are that these lenses seem to dehydrate rather quickly and are incompatible with some solutions.

Classification of soft lens materials

EN ISO 11539:1999 sets out the international standard method for the classification of contact lens materials, and as a published European Standard (EN) it has the status of a British Standard and supersedes those BS classifications in previous use. Each material is classified with a six-part code as shown in Table 2.1.

The Dk range codes are shown in Table 2.2.

As an example, let consider the material netfilcon A III 2. Its classification says that it consists of a polymer with the United States Adopted Names (USAN) prefix net, and that it is a soft lens material (filcon). 'A' indicates that it is the first generation of this polymer, and III that it contains both silicone and fluorine. The number '2' shows its Dk to be between 16 and 30. It is, in fact, the classification for Focus Daily (CIBA).

Table 2.1   Terms used in the ISO system

Prefix	This is administered by USAN and is optional outside the USA. The prefix denotes the polymer used
Stem	This is always filcon for soft lenses, and focon for rigid lenses
Series suffix	Administered by USAN. 'A' indicates the original formulation, 'B' the second vesion, 'C' the third, etc.
Group suffix	I <50% water content, non-ionic II >50% water content, non-ionic III <50% water content, ionic IV >50% water content, ionic
Dk range	A numerical code that identifies the pemeability in ranges. The units are $(cm^2/s.mlO_2)/(s.ml.hPa)$
Modification code	A lower-case letter denoting that the surface has been modified and has different characteristics from the bulk material

Table 2.2   **Oxygen permeability (Dk) ranges**

Group code	Dk range	Examples
1	1–15	All 38% HEMA
2	16–30	All mid/high water content
3	31–60	
4	61–100	
5	101–150	PureVision
		Night and day
6	151–200	
7	200–250	
Higher codes can be added in bands of 50		

Factors influencing water content

The properties of the polymers used in soft contact lenses are dependent on their water content. Any change in that water content will affect the dimensions (i.e. fitting characteristics), surface properties, density, transparency, refractive index and oxygen permeability. The factors that can produce such changes are temperature, tonicity and pH, as well as progressive dehydration during wear.

Between 20°C, which is approximately room temperature, and the on-eye temperature, which is nearer 40°C, there is a drop in water content. The significance of this drop depends on the nature of the material. Group I materials show only a slight effect, but group IV materials are more sensitive. This thermal effect occurs rapidly upon insertion of the lens and is unrelated to the slower, progressive dehydration due to evaporation during wear.

Tonicity may also affect the water content, although the variations encountered in the eye are unlikely to be significant. A change of storage solution may produce a greater effect.

The response to pH is in some respects similar. The variations encountered diurnally in an individual or between individuals are largely insignificant. However, anionic monomers such as MA do react to changes of greater magnitude. Group IV materials, which have both a high water content and anionic components, were unusable at one time, due to the wide range of solutions available in the early 1970s before regulation. They only became a practical proposition as disposable or planned replacement lenses, especially as their anionic groups and large pore size give them a great affinity for lysozyme deposition. Certain peroxide systems have highly acidic pH values, and can cause shrinkage of group IV materials. If insufficient time is allowed for neutralization, the lens may fit tightly following disinfection.

The effects of decreased water content

As the lens loses water, there are significant effects on its dimensions, wettability, friction coefficient and oxygen permeability.

Dimensional stability
The base curve of the lens will generally tighten as the water content reduces. It is widely documented that soft lenses have a short period of 'settling', after which they move rather less than they did on insertion. The settling period is typically about 5 minutes, although with certain lenses and certain patients it can be longer. Temperature-dependent reduction in water content would account for some of this, but thinning of the post-lens tear film associated with initial blinking is also likely to play a part.

Wettability
Hydrogel materials are very wettable when fully hydrated, but as the surface dries, the polymer chains rotate. In contact with

aqueous fluids, the hydrophilic groups are rotated to the surface, but contact with air and lipid will induce those groups to bury themselves, exposing a more hydrophobic surface. The wettability of the material declines throughout the wearing period, and this may account for the high incidence of dry-eye symptoms towards the end of the wearing period. In the fully hydrated state, there is a thin layer of tear fluid between the lens and the cornea, and this tear layer acts as a lubricant. The effect is similar to a car aquaplaning. The frictional properties of the tyre are irrelevant. If this layer breaks down, the frictional properties of the lens surface, rather than the tear film, become important. The result is that the lens will move less freely. At the same time, a reduction in lubrication between the eyelids and the front surface of the lens may increase lid sensation.

Oxygen permeability

There is a simple formula used in membrane science to define the transport of a gas through a polymer membrane:

$$P = DS$$

where P is the permeability coefficient for a given membrane and gas, D is the diffusion coefficient of the gas through that polymer, and S is the solubility of the gas in that polymer.

In the contact lens field, much of the work on oxygen permeability was undertaken by Irving Fatt, who used the term k instead of S. As a result, the contact lens literature uses the term Dk instead of DS or P. Therefore, the permeability coefficient of a contact lens material is its Dk. The actual permeability of a lens will also depend on its thickness. The term used to represent thickness is now t, but in the earlier literature the term L was preferred. Permeability is therefore represented by the term Dk/t, or in older studies Dk/L.

The units of Dk were known as barrer, or more commonly, 'Fatt' units.

$$Dk = 10^{-11} \; (cm^2.mlO_2)/(s.ml.mmHg)$$

Oxygen transmission (Dk/t) in barrer/cm is:

$$Dk/t = 10^{-9} \, (cm^2.mlO_2)/(s.ml.mmHg)$$

However, there is a complication in that the unit mmHg is now internationally obsolete, and the closest accepted metric unit, the hectopascal, is specified in the international standards for contact lenses. Therefore, all Dk values should now be specified in the ISO units, otherwise known as 'New Fatt units'.

The catch is that the new unit is a rather lower Fatt option than the old one, and to convert a Dk value from the old to the new units, the value must be multiplied by a factor of 0.75006. The result is that the Dk is rather less impressive in the new units, and there has been some resistance from the marketing arm of the contact lens industry. Some manufacturers have been quoting in new units, some in old, and some have tried the new ones, found that their rivals were still quoting old values, and gone back to the old system. In time, common sense should prevail, but for the moment it is worth checking the Fatt content of your lenses carefully.

Silicone hydrogel

In 1984, Holden and Mertz found that a minimum oxygen transmissibility of $24 \times 10^{-9} (cm \times ml \, O_2)/(s \times ml \times mmHg)$ was required to avoid clinically detectable signs of edema during daily wear. In extended wear, to limit overnight swelling to less than 4%, a figure of $87 \times 10^{-9} (cm \times ml \, O_2)/(s \times ml \times mmHg)$ was needed. Unfortunately, few of the hydrogel lenses used for daily wear, and none of those used for extended wear, were actually capable of delivering this level of oxygen to the eye. Furthermore, there is wide individual variation in oxygen needs, and the Holden and Mertz figures represent an average figure only. Clearly, something better was needed, especially for extended wear, which became something of an obsession for the industry, although for no particularly obvious commercial reasons at the time. Hydrogel lenses were limited by their reliance on water to transmit the oxygen. If a lens were to have a water content of 100%, it would still fall short of the Holden and Mertz figure for extended wear. The handling and dimensional stability might be less than optimal too, although comfort would be good.

It had been known for some time that silicone rubber is more permeable to oxygen than water, and lenses made from this material have been produced, but silicone rubber is unfortunately hydrophobic. Even with surface treatments, silicone lenses had a tendency to bind to the eye, and removal could be rather difficult. If some way could be found to combine the oxygen permeability of silicone with the hydrophilic properties of hydrogel materials, a lens that both transmitted large quantities of oxygen and moved on the eye might be produced. The obvious solution seemed to be to use the monomer TRIS, which had been successfully used to incorporate silicone into RGP materials. However, TRIS is hydrophobic and HEMA hydrophilic, and combining the two has been likened to mixing oil and water to form an optically clear product. Two approaches were used. The first involved adding polar groups to the TRIS molecule. The second involved macromer technology. Macromers are large monomers that are pre-assembled to give particular properties to the final polymer.

Until 1996, new contact lens materials were evaluated according to their wettability, oxygen permeability and mechanical behavior. A CIBA patent (Griesser et al, 1996) added hydraulic and ion permeability, which determine lens movement on the eye. It described the preparation of a biphasic material with high oxygen and ion permeability, and defined minimum levels of ion or water transmission to allow adequate lens movement on the eye. All subsequent silicone hydrogels exceed these threshold values. The CIBA patent described the material used in Focus Night and Day lenses. Bausch and Lomb released a lens (PureVision) that was essentially homogeneous, although its properties suggest that it may be partially biphasic.

A number of other silicone hydrogel lenses have since emerged, and these are discussed in Chapter 6.

Reference

Griesser HJ, Laycock BG, Papaspiliotopoulos E et al (1996) Extended wear ophthalmic lens. Patent WO 96/31792.

Further reading

Tighe B (2002) Soft lens materials. In: Efron N (ed.) *Contact Lens Practice*, pp 71–84. Butterworth-Heinmann: Oxford.

3
Spherical lens fitting

Introduction   36
Initial measurements   36
The principles of soft lens fitting   37
Modality   40
Handling soft lenses   41
    Removal of a soft lens   48
Assessing the fit   50
References   56

Introduction

Once we have established that the patient is suitable for soft
lenses, we can proceed to selecting the initial trial lens. Most soft
lenses used in practice these days are selected from banks of
lenses covering the common range of powers and fits available in
the range. This is possible because most spherical lenses are only
available in one total diameter and one or two radii, which would
seem to make soft lens selection and fitting a very simple affair.
Sadly, this is not the case.

Initial measurements

There are several measurements that students of optometry are
usually trained to perform, and it is worth considering what they
contribute to the selection process for soft lenses.

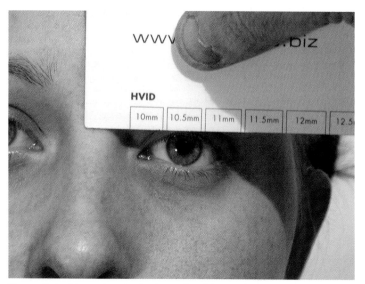

Figure 3.1 Measuring the horizontal visible iris diameter

The **horizontal visible iris diameter** (HVID) is usually measured with a ruler (Fig. 3.1), but greater accuracy can be achieved by using a measuring graticule on a slit-lamp, thus eliminating parallax errors. The main point is to decide whether to fit a large-diameter lens or a small-diameter one.

The **visible palpebral aperture** (VPA) has little relevance to a soft lens, although a small VPA, especially if paired with tight lids, as it usually is, might encourage the use of a smaller-diameter lens, if only to aid insertion and removal.

There is usually little point in measuring **pupil diameters**, unless the patient is highly ametropic or multifocal lenses are under consideration, as soft lenses have relatively large optic zones and rarely, if ever, suffer from 'flare'. The extent of front surface lenticulation required for very high-powered soft lenses may result in some flare if the patient has large pupils. Some multifocal lenses will perform indifferently with the wrong-sized pupils (see Chapter 6).

The principles of soft lens fitting

The goal of soft lens fitting is to pair the primary sag of the back surface of the lens optimally with that of the front surface of the eye. If the latter were a simple spherical surface, the task would be easy. However, the cornea is known to be aspheric in nature. In most people, it can be described as a prolate ellipse (Guillon and Ho, 1994). That is, it flattens towards the periphery. The degree of flattening (asphericity) can be expressed in terms of 'eccentricity' or as a 'shape factor'. The average eccentricity for the human cornea is 0.39, which correlates with a shape factor of 0.85. The problem is that it does not always flatten at the same rate, as shape factors vary between +0.50 and −0.10. A negative value indicates a cornea that steepens peripherally, which occurs in about 3% of the population. There is little correlation between the rate of flattening and the values found by keratometry. Two eyes with the same K reading can have widely differing rates of flattening, even in the same individual. The rates may be different horizontally and vertically. Modern topographic studies have identified five groups:

- round (23% symmetric, very low astigmatism)
- oval (21% asymmetric, very low astigmatism)
- symmetric bow-tie (17.5% symmetric astigmatic)
- asymmetric bow-tie (32% asymmetric astigmatic)
- irregular (7%, no pattern).

This is complicated enough, but a soft lens will also overlap the cornea and cover the limbus and part of the scleral conjunctiva, which is rather flatter than the cornea. The back surface of a soft lens is flatter than the central area of the cornea but steeper than the peripheral cornea and scleral conjunctiva. A flexible contact lens will distort in order to align with the underlying curvature, so the lens steepens in the center and flattens in the periphery. The forces generated within the lens by this distortion create 'squeeze pressure', which acts on the tear film and the eye. It is this squeeze pressure that seems to determine how a soft lens fits and moves on the eye. The art of fitting soft lenses is largely one of manipulating this squeeze pressure, and as yet it remains an art rather than an exact science.

   To tighten or loosen the fit, intuition leads the practitioner to the conclusion that if the back optic zone radius (BOZR) is steeper, the lens will fit tighter, and this has been the traditional approach to initial lens selection for much of the history of the soft lens. Most students of optometry have learned the hoary old rule of thumb and dutifully add 0.6/1.00 mm to average/flatten K. However, the fact that there are several versions of this rule of thumb might suggest that none of them actually works very well, and there is research to support that view. Even with fairly thick low-water-content lenses, Lowther and Tomlinson (1981) found that a large change in BOZR was required to produce any detectable change in lens movement, and with the thinner, higher-water-content lenses in use currently, there is even less effect. Young (1992) has shown that corneal sagittal height is more dependent on individual variations in corneal shape factor than on the normal distribution of K readings. Flatter corneas tend to be larger in diameter, so if the shape factor was to remain constant, the effect of increasing radius, which would reduce the sag, would be offset by the effect of an increased diameter, which would increase it. If asphericity is the critical variant, this might suggest that photokeratoscopic mapping could be a fruitful area of study with regard to soft lens design. However, this has not yet been adopted in optometric practice to any extent.

As if the topography of the eye and the flexure of the lens are not enough to contend with, there are several variables that the lens design itself will introduce. It is widely accepted that lenses of different brands with apparently similar parameters behave rather differently on the eye, and not always predictably.

- Total diameter. Intuitively, you would expect a bigger lens to move rather less than a small one on a given eye, since the lens is overlapping a greater area of flatter scleral conjunctiva. On the whole, this is true, but not always, as other aspects of the lens design may influence the squeeze pressure that the lens develops. Some manufacturers make their plus lenses with a bigger total diameter in an attempt to reduce the greater movement expected. However, given that most hyperopes tend to have smaller-diameter corneas, this may be of limited benefit.

The flexibility of the lens or of areas of the lens will be affected by a number of factors.

- Center thickness. The thinner the lens, the more oxygen it will transmit. However, below a certain point, the lens becomes over-susceptible to dehydration, and handling becomes difficult. Therefore, mid-water lenses are generally made with a center thickness in the 0.06–0.10 mm range. High-water-content lenses have to be made thicker, and are typically 0.10–0.18 in the center.
- Back vertex power. The average thickness of the lens, and the thickness at a point away from the center, will increase with increasing back vertex power. For minus lenses, up to about −1.50 diopter (D), the center thickness is usually

increased a little to improve handling. High-minus lenses also tend to have a smaller optic zone and a reduced center thickness. The use of aspheric optics can also allow a high-minus lens to be made thinner, while at the same time improving visual performance by correcting spherical aberration, provided that the lens centers well. Plus lenses also usually have reduced optic zones. The actual effect of back vertex power on movement is limited over the usual range of minus lenses, but plus lenses are generally thought to move more than minus types of the same design.

- Edge thickness may significantly affect lens movement, although not always in the way expected. Young found that lenses with a thicker edge often seemed to fit looser than similar lenses with a thinner edge. Edge thickness is partly a function of the method of manufacture of the lens. Molded lenses can be made with very thin edges, whereas lathe-cut lenses need thicker edges to survive the manufacturing process. However, lenses with thin edges may be difficult to handle, so some lenses are made with thicker edges to avoid this problem.

Modality

The soft lenses currently available commercially can be divided into a number of categories defined by the expected working life of the lens.

Daily disposable lenses are intended to be worn once, and then discarded.

Planned replacement lenses are replaced at rather longer intervals, typically either 2 weeks (in the USA) or 1 month (in Europe). The replacement interval is influenced by economic as much as clinical considerations, being linked to the frequency of salary payments typical in the respective continents.

What used to be called '**conventional**' lenses are now anything but that, and tend to be used only when there is no planned replacement alternative. They are usually replaced at 6-monthly or yearly intervals.

There are several advantages to a short contact lens working life:

- The fewer times the lens has to survive handling and cleaning, the flimsier it can be. This allows it to be thinner, so it can transmit more oxygen.
- Lenses made to be replaced frequently have less opportunity to collect deposits, so the use of group IV materials is practical. This makes mass manufacture commercially viable.
- Fewer deposits mean less chair time dealing with allergic and inflammatory reactions to them.
- The need to obtain a new pack of lenses every so often can help with compliance with aftercare, although this is somewhat compromised if the patient obtains their lenses from an internet-based supplier.
- Frequent replacement lenses need specific protein cleaners only rarely, especially with modern multipurpose solutions. Daily disposables need no disinfection either.

The choice of modality will depend on patient preference, bearing in mind their specific visual and physiologic requirements. On the whole, daily disposable lenses are a little more expensive, but more convenient. On the other hand, monthly lenses are available in a wider range of parameters and materials, including useful toric, multifocal and flexible wear options.

Handling soft lenses

Patients are generally rather nervous around optometrists. There has been research showing that people are more stressed when having a sight test than during a dental appointment. Contact lens patients have the added stress of allowing someone to invade their personal space and stick a bit of plastic in their eye. The eye has a sophisticated defense mechanism to prevent things entering it. It is therefore important that the practitioner projects a calm demeanor, and avoids words such as 'pain'. Like politicians, we must sweeten the pill, and emphasize the immediate comfort likely to be experienced. This might not be absolutely true, but the best time to point out that the saline in which the lens has been stored might cause a tiny bit of stinging is probably when the lens is already in the eye, settling. It is essential that the practitioner be a source of calm and confidence. This is much easier to achieve if the practitioner is actually calm and confident, and competence in the handling of lenses will calm the nerves of both parties. The only way to achieve competence is by practice, but a little bit of technique can help as well.

Before a patient is touched, thorough washing of the hands should occur, preferably in clear sight of the patient. In addition to the obvious antimicrobial benefits, this will serve to reassure the patient that they are in good (or at least clean) hands, and it may influence their own approach to lens hygiene. Cold water may be best for the final rinsing, as rising mains water is less likely to contain *Acanthamoeba*.

When handling soft lenses, we must take a number of lens characteristics into account. Soft lenses are rather large compared to rigid gas permeable (RGP) lenses, and one of the challenges is therefore how to get something that size into the typical human palpebral aperture. Soft lenses are also quite soft, as the name might indicate. Some of the thinner ones are downright floppy, until they lose some water. They then distort and take on some of the characteristics of thin potato crisps, although they are possibly less comfortable on the eye. Also, it is easily possible to turn them inside out, and to insert them into the patient's eye in this state.

It follows, therefore, that our insertion technique should allow us to deliver a lens the right way round and reasonably hydrated to the right part of the eye without alarming the patient unduly, or needing to apply unreasonable force to any bit of them. First, we need to check that the lens is not inside out. Some lenses have markings on them that a sharp-eyed pre-presbyope, in good lighting, or on a slit-lamp, might be able to see. For the most part, however, we need to do the following. Place the lens on the end of a finger and observe it from the side. The typical appearance of lenses the correct and wrong

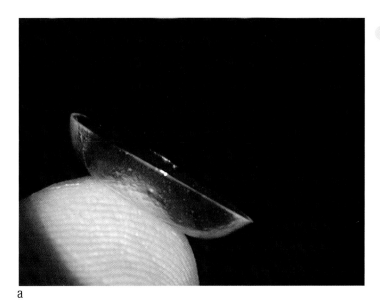

a

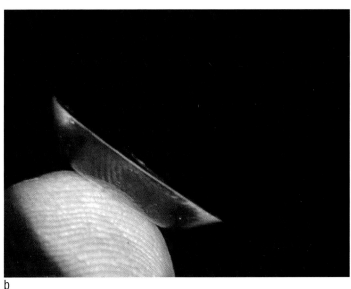

b

Figure 3.2 (a) Lens correct way round. (b) Lens inside out

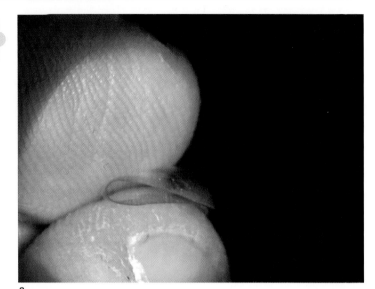

a

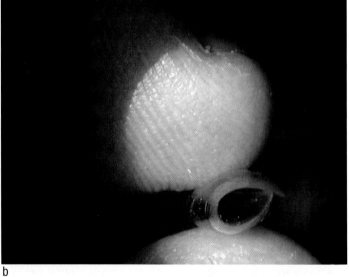

b

Figure 3.3 Pinching a lens – it easily folds if the correct way round. (a) Lens incorrect way round when pinched. (b) Lens correct way round when pinched

ways round can be seen in Figure 3.2. Next, pinch the lens as shown in Figure 3.3. A lens the correct way round will fold inwards easily. A lens that is inside out will resist, and try to fold back on your fingers.

The next challenge to address is that of finding enough room to insert the lens. In general, this is best done by directing the patient to look to their left when inserting a lens into the right eye (and to their right when inserting a lens into the left eye) and either downwards or upwards (Fig. 3.4).

The lens is applied to the temporal sclera, and centered on the cornea afterwards. If the patient's head is tilted back on the headrest, looking down and in will give the biggest target area on most people, as the upper lid can be pulled back further than the lower one. However, in many patients, looking up and in will give a perfectly adequate target area and has the additional advantage with a nervous patient of allowing for Bell's phenomenon, where attempted reflex closure of the lids is accompanied by upward rolling of the eyes to protect the cornea. There are also some soft lenses that are 'heavy' and tend to fall off the finger if the eye

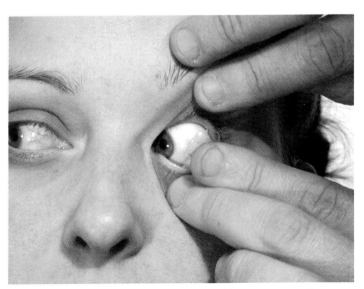

Figure 3.4 Ensure as large a surface as possible prior to insertion

is approached from on high. The up-and-under approach works best for these. Ideally, a practitioner should be able to switch between techniques according to individual requirements. In either case, the lids must be controlled. The upper lid is often best controlled by a thumb placed near the lid margin, which should allow sufficient control to be exerted without causing discomfort to the patient. The lower lid is generally controlled by the finger next to that bearing the lens. Most students put the lens on the first finger for their early attempts at lens insertion, but for many practitioners the middle finger is longer. If the lens is placed on the end of this finger, the extra length may allow some bending of the finger, which may assist insertion. Whichever finger is used, the lens should be placed on the tip, so that the area of contact between the finger and the lens surface is minimal. This makes it easier for the tear film to pull the lens from the finger. The approach to the eye should not be too slow. The longer it goes on, the more likely the patient is to lose their nerve. The lens may dry out as well, especially on a hot day, and it may then be reluctant to leave your finger.

The technique for applying the lens to the eye is a little different from that used for RGP lenses. In the latter case, one merely has to touch the lens to the eye and the tear film will claim the lens. With a soft lens, the lens must be squashed gently onto the surface of the sclera, and it may help to slightly roll the finger. This will help to dispel any air pockets under the lens and help the lens to part from the finger. At this point we have a lens sitting on the upper or lower temporal sclera, probably a bit wrinkled and vulnerable to a sudden blink. It is important to retain control of the lids at this stage, while directing the patient to look towards the lens, then up, down, etc. until the lens is centered on the cornea and most of the air expelled. We can then gently let the lids go.

Usually, a soft lens is comfortable from the start. If it is not, there are a number of possibilities.

- The saline that lenses are stored in becomes progressively acidic over time. If a lens has been in the bank for a long time,

it may take a few seconds for the pH to normalize, and the lenses may sting a little on insertion.
- The lens may be damaged.
- There may be a foreign body trapped under the lens.
- There may be an air bubble.

If the saline is causing the discomfort, it will pass in a few moments. If the patient can manage it, have a look on the slit-lamp. If not, remove the lens, clean and rinse it thoroughly, and re-insert it, provided that the eye is not damaged. During professional examinations, candidates are sometimes observed massaging a newly inserted lens vigorously through the lids to clear trapped air. This is both unnecessary, as trapped air will usually find a way out unaided, and dangerous, as any foreign body under the lens will create spirograph patterns in the corneal epithelium and provide a potential source of entry for microbes.

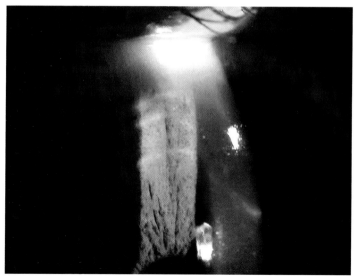

Figure 3.5 Abrasion of the cornea due to poor handling

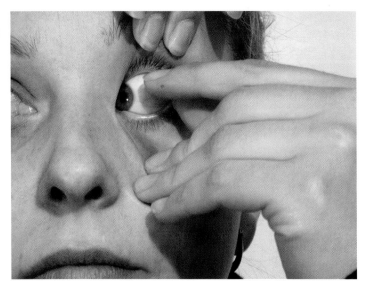

Figure 3.6 Removal of a soft lens

Removal of a soft lens

It is generally not a good idea for the practitioner to attempt removal of a soft lens directly from the cornea. A heavy-handed approach might lead to mechanical abrasion of the cornea (Fig. 3.5), similar to that sometimes seen at aftercare visits.

The technique usually favored is essentially the reverse of insertion. The lens is decentered temporally using a finger, and then the thumb is brought in to pinch the lens off the surface of the sclera (Fig. 3.6).

Usually, the upper lid needs to be pulled out of the way with a thumb or finger, and the lower lid may need to be controlled.

An alternative is a version of the common RGP lens removal technique, where the lens is pinched out between the two lids, in this case direct from the cornea. The patient needs to have a wide palpebral aperture, as soft lenses are rather larger than RGP lenses, and the flexibility of the lens is also important. This method works best with 'stiffer' lenses such as silicone hydrogel and some toric lenses.

Occasionally, a patient will panic and develop blepharospasm. This can make removal of the lens impossible. Fortunately, there is a trick that almost always works. In a calm, confident tone of voice, tell the patient the following: 'When I say go, open your mouth as far as you can. GO!' It is almost impossible to close the lids tightly and open the mouth wide at the same time. Also, the drawing of attention towards the mouth, away from the eye, may contribute to the effect. In any case, it will usually give you enough time to get the lens out.

If a lens is immobile, the practitioner should not attempt to take it out without irrigating the eye first. It is possible that there is little or no post-lens tear film present, and the lens may be binding to the cornea. If the lens is removed in this state, it may take some of the epithelium with it. Irrigation can be a messy business, but the use of single-dose saline is hygienic and may limit leakage. The usual technique is to apply a generous quantity

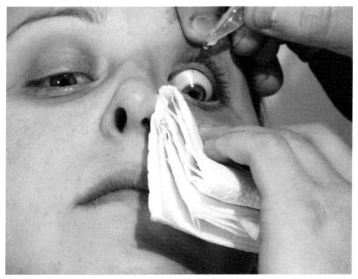

Figure 3.7 Irrigating an eye

of paper towels to the side of the face below the eye to catch the excess (Fig. 3.7).

It sometimes happens that the lens goes in and then disappears. It is not where it should be, but it has not exited the eye either. In this case, evert the lids, as thin lenses do have a habit of hiding under the top one, and try instilling fluorescein, as it will stain a soft lens and make it more apparent. This is also a useful technique when looking for lens fragments. Irrigation of the eye may also be required. Occasionally, a lens will roll itself up and move well into the upper fornix. If the usual search is fruitless, ask the patient to come back the next day. The lens cannot do much harm up there in the short term, and it will probably work its way out in time.

Assessing the fit

The first question to address is how long the lens will take to settle. It has become traditional in practice to allow 20 minutes. This is remarkably similar to the span allocated to a standard appointment, or in quieter periods to drink a cup of your favorite beverage. Brennan has pointed out that most soft lenses do most of their settling in the first 2 minutes, and it is widely accepted that the fit after 5 minutes probably is not going to change much for several hours. Over this initial period, there is some dispute about exactly what is happening. The temperature of the lens will rise on the eye, the water content will fall, and the fit will tighten to some extent. However, these changes probably only account for part of the settling process. It is likely that the lens initially traps a thick tear film under it, which is then squeezed out by some complementary blinking. However it occurs, the net effect is that the lens will move less after 5 minutes than it did upon insertion, unless, that is, the practitioner inadvertently muddies the waters. This is actually not that hard to do, or that uncommon. The way to do this is to shine a bright light into the patient's eye and fiddle obsessively with the lens. If you irritate the eye sufficiently, even the most limpet-like hydrogel lens can be prodded into respectable movement. This is important, because for a soft lens, movement is crucial.

If the lens were entirely static on the eye, the parts of the cornea under the thickest parts of the lens would always receive less oxygen than those under thinner areas. Given that hydrogel materials are not exactly over-generous with their oxygen transmission, this means that in many patients a part of the cornea would be too hypoxic for continued health. In the case of a myope, the thickest part of the lens would probably lie over an area just inside the limbus. The distressed epithelial cells would therefore be ideally placed to release chemical stimuli to the limbal vessels, which would then start to grow.

The epithelial cells are constantly being replaced, and the dead upper layer is sloughed off in the tear film. A soft contact lens will tend to prevent the efficient clearing of such debris, and indeed of other material trapped under the lens. This trapped material may act as a stimulus to inflammatory events, particularly in extended wear situations. It is hardly surprising, then, that immobile lenses have been linked to inflammatory events, neovascularization and microbial keratitis.

To summarize, then, movement is a good thing. However, you can have too much of a good thing, but what does too much look like? There are various numbers bandied about, but none of them really means much. We need to look at the practicalities. If the lens moves a lot, what are the problems?

1. The patient will not be able to see properly, which rather defeats the object of the exercise. A loose lens will give the patient unstable vision, which typically only clears immediately after a blink. Furthermore, if the patient is wearing two lenses of substantial power that are moving rather randomly, some interesting prismatic effects may be generated.
2. The lens will probably be uncomfortable, as the edge is probably wrinkling, and the lens is interacting with the lids more than intended.
3. The lens will probably be crossing the limbus during the blink cycle. In most cases, this will result in drying and localized

epithelial damage, which in turn increases the chances of inflammation or infection. However, it is not unknown to see patients at aftercare whose lenses cross the limbus without any detectable physiologic effect. In these cases, no action is needed.

4. There does appear to be a link between loose lenses and contact lens-related papillary conjunctivitis (CLPC), particularly when the stiffer silicone hydrogel lenses are worn. However, if a lens does induce CLPC mechanically, tightening the fit or fitting a less stiff lens will usually solve the problem.

In general, a lens that is too loose and mobile will manifest as an unhappy patient. If the patient is happy with the vision and comfort, and the movement is not causing problems due to exposure at the limbus, the fit is a good one.

We now need to consider what a lens that is not too loose looks like. In general, unless they are grossly tight, most lenses will move slightly when the patient blinks or the eyes undertake excursions, so most practitioners will observe the lens in these situations in some variation of the following sequence.

1. With the patient looking straight ahead, observe the movement of the lens with a blink. This is often rather small with modern lenses. It is often useful to reduce the braking effect of the eyelids by directing the patient to look up a little. A well-fitting lens will often move about 0.5 mm in this position, but may move more or less. Occasionally, you may need to raise a tight upper lid as well. The 'sag' (downwards decentration) of the lens and the movement with a blink should be recorded as fractions of a millimeter rather than in subjective terms such as 'good'. Our concept of good can alter over the years. The accurate recording of movement is difficult to master at first, although it becomes easier with practice, and overestimation is the norm. Measurement with an eyepiece graticule, or a graduated slit height or width, may make things easier, but the most common technique is to compare the amplitude of any movement with the overlap of

the lens over the limbus. If we know the HVID, and the total diameter of the lens, we can easily work this out. The value is typically 0.75–1.5 mm. The technique of comparison is also useful when recording vessel growth.

2. The 'lag' of the lens when the eye moves to the left and right can be recorded in the same way. Lag and sag tend to be highest in thicker, stiffer, heavier lenses, and older texts tend to afford these qualities rather more importance than they warrant when assessing modern hydrogel lenses.

3. Because many modern lenses do not show much lag and sag, the **push-up test** is important, although its use seems shrouded in mystery. If the lens is showing plenty of lag and sag, it is largely a waste of time, as we already know the lens to be freely mobile. However, if a lens is not sagging and lagging, there could be a number of explanations.

   (a) The lens could be tight, exerting undue squeeze pressure on the limbus and sclera. Very tight fits tend to result in unstable vision, with loss of clarity after a blink, and in perilimbal flush after a while. However, slightly tight fits look rather like optimal ones, until the lens eventually stops moving.

   (b) The post-lens tear film could have been squeezed out, or it could have dried out.

   (c) The lens is thin and light, and gravity is having little effect on it.

   (d) The lids are unable to get sufficient purchase on the slick lens surface to move the lens when blinking.

   (e) The lids are acting as a brake, restricting lens movement.

The push-up test separates the first two possibilities, which have potential to damage the eye, from the rest.

The test is conducted by using the thumb on the patient's lower lid to push the lower edge of lens upwards (Fig. 3.8).

The squeeze pressure that the lens is exerting can be gauged from both the force required to move the lens upwards, and the speed of recovery to a central position. The force that is applied can be recorded in a number of ways, but some sort of numerical or percentage scale is useful, as it may allow comparisons after

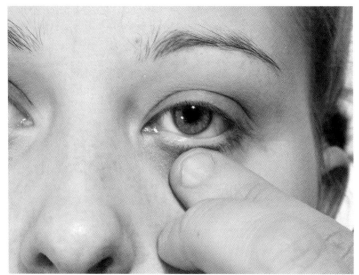

a

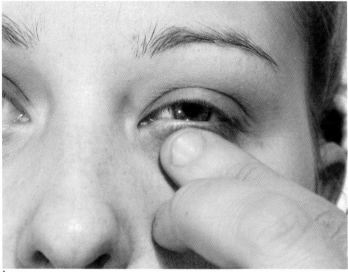

b

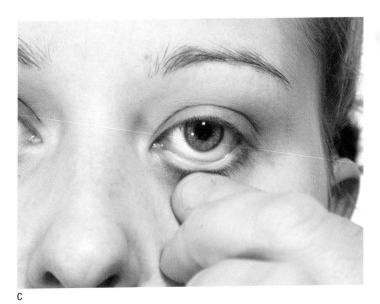

C

Figure 3.8 Push-up test

different wearing periods. Some practitioners use a percentage scale that starts at 50% for an optimal lens, whereas others denote a freely moving lens as 0% or simply 0. In the absence of any internationally recognized system, use one that is intuitive to you.

The recovery can also be numerated, but is more frequently described as 'rapid', 'medium' or 'slow'.

Because of the subjective nature of gauging a lens with your thumb, the exact point at which a lens feels too tight is also somewhat intuitive. However, on the whole, provided that the lens is not loose enough to irritate the patient, most practitioners are happiest with a lens that requires little or no effort to move.

This is because soft lenses lose water through evaporation throughout the period of wear. As discussed in Chapter 2, this can reduce oxygen transmission and wettability, and the dimensions of the lens will change. The fit will generally tighten, especially on a minus-powered lens. The speed at which this process occurs will depend upon the lens material, the tear characteristics of the patient, and the temperature and humidity of the environment, but it is usually measurable in hours rather than minutes. A lens that is freely mobile at the start of the wearing period has a better chance of staying mobile throughout wear, on a long, hot day. A lens that requires significant effort to move after 5 minutes is likely to develop limpet-like tendencies after a few hours of wear. The 'feel' of a good lens is one of those skills that develops with practice and experience, but if in doubt it is a wise precaution to conduct an extended trial with the lens, by inserting the lens in the morning, and reassessing towards the end of the day. This can be conducted as part of the initial fitting itself, but should be part of the aftercare sequence even for lenses that you expect to be beyond reproach. Ocular topography being what it is, making too many assumptions about a contact lens fit is asking for trouble. It is always best to check.

References

Guillon M and Ho A (1994) Photokeratoscopy. In: Ruben M and Guillon M (eds) *Contact Lens Practice*, pp 313–357. Chapman & Hall Medical, Oxford.

Lowther G and Tomlinson A (1981) Critical base curve and diameter interval in the fitting of spherical soft contact lenses. *Am J Optom* **58**: 355–360.

Young G (1992) Ocular sagittal height and soft contact lens fit. *J Br Contact Lens Assoc* **15**: 45–49.

4
Soft lenses for astigmatism

Introduction   58
Aspheric lenses   59
Fitting soft toric lenses   59
Measuring lens rotation   60
Stabilization   62
Troubleshooting   65
  Poor vision   65
  Poor comfort   66
  Hypoxia   67
  Staining   67

Introduction

A soft contact lens will attempt to align itself with the contours of the eye that it sits upon. If the corneal surface is astigmatic, the lens will conform to that astigmatic surface. It used to be thought that a soft lens could mask a certain amount of astigmatism, especially a thick one, but although this may have been true for the very early, thick, low-water-content lenses originally in use, it is certainly not the case for modern lenses. A spherical soft lens will not correct any useful amount of corneal astigmatism. However, some astigmatic individuals may see slightly better with a thick soft lens, at the considerable cost of reduced oxygen transmission and increased physiologic compromise.

Patients may tolerate a certain amount of uncorrected astigmatism, particularly if the lenses are worn for visually undemanding tasks. Those who wear lenses for sports or social reasons may put up with a surprising amount of visual compromise if motivation is high. However, tolerance to blur does vary between patients, and for visually demanding tasks uncorrected astigmatism may be unacceptable. In general, any patient with residual astigmatism over 0.75D should be offered the option of a toric lens if their visual needs are likely to warrant it. Approximately one-third of the population fall into this category, and about 7% have astigmatism over 2.00D. Oddly, less than 20% of soft lenses fitted are toric, although this figure is rising year by year. Practitioner reluctance to recommend them to patients has probably been a factor, for historical reasons.

Not so long ago, toric soft lenses did not enjoy a good reputation. Indeed, the poor levels of reproducibility led to them being known in some circles as 'snowflakes', as you could never get two the same. In those days, rigid gas permeable (RGP) lenses were the first choice for correcting astigmatism, but the past decade has seen the emergence of reliable, easily fitted toric soft lenses, which have eroded the RGP lens market significantly. It is now possible to fit toric lenses for all wearing modalities, even (to a limited extent) daily wear. Silicone hydrogel toric lenses are available, and even toric multifocal lenses can be found. As a result, soft toric lenses are usually the first choice for an astigmatic patient.

Aspheric lenses

Some soft lens designs incorporate an aspheric front surface to correct the eye's spherical aberration, and it has been claimed that they can give good acuity in astigmatism up to 1.50D by reducing the blur circle. There does seem to be quite a lot of variation between individuals, but this type of lens is worth considering for low degrees of astigmatism. They are simple to fit and require no stabilization system, as they have no axis to stabilize. The availability of reliable soft toric lenses has tended to make them less popular.

Fitting soft toric lenses

The requirements for a good fit are the same for a toric lens as for a spherical one, so the movement on blink, lag, sag and response to push-up test will also be the same. A lens that is too tight will not rotate properly, and the astigmatic correction will not align along the desired meridian. It may rotate progressively as the lower lid spins it and be too immobile to recover, so a lens where the reference marks are some way off their expected position should be regarded with suspicion. Those that are too loose will probably spin around randomly. A well-fitting lens should enable the various stabilization systems to work to keep the lens on axis.

Toric lenses generally have engraved lines along their nominal horizontal and/or vertical meridians to indicate how much the lens has rotated on the eye. This enables the practitioner to offset the astigmatic axis so that when the lens is on the eye, the optical correction is accurate. For example, consider the following spectacle prescription:

PLANO/−2.00 × 80

If the reference lines on the lens are seen to rotate by 10° in a clockwise direction, the cylinder on the eye would have an axis of 70°. We therefore need to change the prescription of the lens to:

PLANO/−2.00 × 90

This will ensure that the axis will align correctly once the lens takes up its habitual rotated position.

- **Clockwise** rotation of the lens needs to be **added** to the axis.
- **Anticlockwise** rotation need to be **subtracted**.

This gives Clockwise Add, Anticlockwise Subtract, or CAAS.
A common variation of the above rule is the 'LARS' rule. This concept relies on the fact that most of the reference marks are found in the vertical meridian on the lower part of the lens.

- Clockwise rotation of the lens causes the reference line to move **left** and we need to **add** the rotation to the axis.
- Anticlockwise rotation causes the reference line to move **right** and we must **subtract** the rotation from the axis.

To summarize, the rule is Left Add, Right Subtract, or LARS.

Measuring lens rotation

Before we add or subtract anything, it would be a good idea to measure the lens rotation on the eye. Lenses use a variety of markings to indicate orientation (Fig. 4.1).

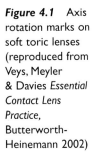

Figure 4.1 Axis rotation marks on soft toric lenses (reproduced from Veys, Meyler & Davies *Essential Contact Lens Practice,* Butterworth-Heinemann 2002)

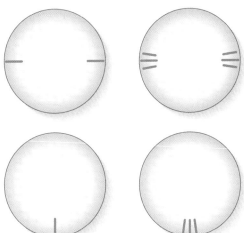

A number of methods may be used:

1. An **eyepiece graticule** calibrated in degrees may be used on the slit-lamp.
2. A thin **slit-lamp beam** may be rotated to align with the reference lines on the lens if there is a suitable scale on the slit-lamp illumination system. Alternatively, some focusing rods are calibrated in degrees and the alignment of the beam can be measured from this.
3. Sphero-cylindrical over-refraction (SCO) may be undertaken with the lens inserted and settled. Torics tend to take longer than spherical lenses to settle, so an extended trial may be useful here, especially if the cylindrical content is large and accuracy at a premium. The spectacle prescription, trial lens power and over-refraction can be put into a programmable calculator or computer to determine the final power; the software for this is widely available from manufacturers. Alternatively, the trial contact lens power and over-refraction may be placed in a trial frame and neutralized with a focimeter (lensmeter). This is the most accurate way to determine the power and axis, and should certainly be the method of choice

if one is faced with an extremely expensive custom lens with a high astigmatic power.

4. The most common method used for lower powers is '**guesstimation**'. Optometrists, through practice, become rather good at estimating angles, and manufacturers often provide useful extra reference lines either side of the main one, at intervals of 10° or 15°. Many disposable lenses are only available with axes at 10° intervals anyway, so this method is accurate enough in most cases.

5. If you are fitting daily toric lenses, it is even simpler; at present, they are only available with axis of 90° or 180°, so you pick the nearest and hope.

Stabilization

Having taken the trouble to measure and calculate the axis, you do not want the lens to rotate at random, which, left to its own devices, it might. During the blink cycle, closure of the lids proceeds from the outer to inner canthus ('the zipper effect'). The upper lid moves vertically down to close the eye, and then up again to open it. The lower lid, however, does not move vertically, so as it tightens it imparts a force on the lens that will tend to spin the lower part of the lens nasally. Some cyclorotation of the eye may also play a part. To counteract this tendency, several strategies are employed.

1. **Back surface toricity** is intended to align the lens more exactly with the cornea. However, although this is undoubtedly effective when applied to RGP lenses, it is of questionable effectiveness with modern, flexible soft lenses, since they all tend to conform to the underlying surface. It is always used with other stabilization methods. Any effect that it has is likely to be greatest where the corneal astigmatism is high. Most disposable toric lenses have this feature.

2. **Prism ballast** is commonly used. The lower lens edge is thickened. When the eyes close during the blink cycle, the squeeze pressure imparted by the upper lid impels the thickest

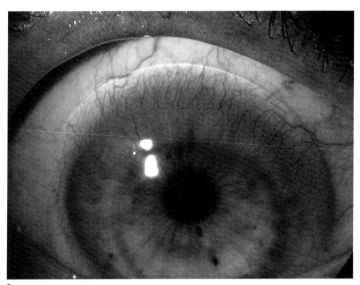

a

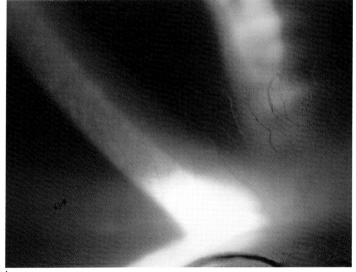

b

Figure 4.2 (a) Limbal neovascularization. (b) Ghost vessels, alongside some containing blood, in a toric soft lens wearer

part of the lens away. This is known as the 'watermelon seed principle'. Prism ballast is effective, but it has the disadvantage of adding thickness to the lens in the area of the lower limbus. This will reduce oxygen transmission, and when low-water-content lenses were commonly fitted, this often led to hypoxia and subsequent neovascularization of the lower cornea (Figure 4.2).

3. In addition, vertical prismatic effect may be induced, although this effect is only likely to be about one-third of the incorporated prism, and patient intolerance due to it is rare. Modern lenses may have an optic zone without prism.

4. **Truncation** is occasionally used in conjunction with prism ballast. Effectively, this consists of chopping off part of the lower lens periphery so that the lower lens edge is straight or has a greater radius than the rest of the lens.

5. **Dynamic stabilization** (thin zone stabilization) also uses the watermelon seed principle, but here material is removed from both the upper and lower lens edges, so both lids contribute to the stabilizing effect. The lenses have thin edges, so they tend to be a little more comfortable, and no prismatic effect is induced. Some practitioners prefer them for against-the-rule astigmatism, as they tend to thin down the areas of the lens that the cylinder would render thickest. However, prism ballast may give a slightly better visual performance post-blink. The earlier dynamically stabilized lenses had the disadvantage that the thickness differential was dependent on power, with greater stabilizing effect with increasing minus. This has been addressed by designs with a central optic zone and a separately worked peripheral area containing the thin zones. This allows greater consistency of response across the power range and controls the thickness profile and oxygen transmission of the higher-minus lenses. A variation on the dynamic stabilization theme is the incorporation of shaped, raised areas in the horizontal meridian of a lenticulated lens. This will also allow a thin edge, although the raised areas may cause lid sensation.

6. **Lenticulation, chamfer** and **slab-off** on the front surface of the lens may all be used to thin the edges and improve comfort. When combined with prism ballast, the idea is to

produce a more uniform edge thickness. '**Eccentric lenticulation**' produces a zone decentered upwards, to reduce the influence of the lower lid.

The geometry of modern lenses has become quite complex in the quest to combine lens stability with comfort and oxygen transmission, and the lenses in use today are far more sophisticated and effective than the 'snowflakes' of former times.

Troubleshooting

Soft toric lens fitting is usually fairly straightforward these days, but not quite as straightforward as spherical fitting. Studies have shown that an average of 1.5–1.8 lenses per eye is required to achieve a satisfactory result for soft toric lenses. Sensible practitioners will manage patient expectations before commencing the fitting process, so that having to reorder lenses is not perceived as professional incompetence. If the patient is prepared for a certain amount of difficulty, you may get lucky with the first pair of lenses. The patient will then see you as a paragon of optometric skill, which will do your practice no harm at all. Common problems that may arise include reduced or unstable vision, poor comfort, hypoxia and staining.

Poor vision

If the visual result is disappointing, we need to determine whether it is constantly or variable poor.

Constant poor vision may be associated with the following:

1. wrong powers for spherical or astigmatic components
2. mislocation of axis (more probable)
3. both power and axis are wrong.

A spectacle over-refraction should give an indication of the remedy, although axis mislocation can also be detected by observation with a slit-lamp as outlined earlier in this chapter.

Axis mislocation produces a characteristic type of residual refractive error. The cylindrical power is twice that of the spherical component, and the axis moves in the same direction of rotation as that of the mislocating lens. For example a lens of $-2.75/1.50 \times 180$ that has rotated $20°$ anticlockwise will have an over-refraction of $+0.50/-1.00 \times 55$. Crossed cylinder calculation can be used to remedy the correction. This is often performed by the laboratory, but can be done by the practitioner if preferred.

Occasionally, every change to the lens axis to remedy mislocation results in the new lens rotating by a different amount, because the thickness profile of the lens has changed. This is called '**chasing the axis**', and is normally associated with large cylindrical elements, oblique axes, and older designs. Use of a design with independent optic and peripheral zones may help, although the usual remedy to this in practice is a lucky guess.

Unstable vision may be caused by a steep or flat-fitting lens:

1. Steep lenses tend to flex irregularly, so the vision often improves just after a blink, and then deteriorates. The axis may also slowly rotate in one direction with successive blinks.
2. Flat lenses may rotate randomly.

If the fit of the lens looks good, but the vision is unstable, the stabilization systems incorporated in the design may not be working for this patient, so another type of design may be better. It is always a good idea to have a favorite prism-ballasted lens and a favorite dynamically stabilized one to try in these circumstances.

Some patients simply do not like the visual quality afforded by soft lenses. They may be happier with RGP lenses, but there are those who can accept no visual compromise. They will probably never be happy with any sort of lens.

Poor comfort

Toric lenses tend to be thicker than spherical ones around the edges, particularly if they have prism ballast or truncation. For this reason, they may be less comfortable than the spherical

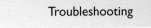

equivalent. Where comfort is an issue, the aim should be to use as thin a lens as possible. Dynamically stabilized designs tend to be useful here.

Hypoxia

Toric lenses are generally thicker than the equivalent spherical lenses, and this will reduce their oxygen transmission, at least in some locations under the lens. In earlier times, low-water-content hydroxyethylmethacrylate (HEMA) lenses with prism ballast became somewhat notorious for causing edema and considerable neovascularization of the lower cornea. With modern designs, there is less of a problem, but it should still be kept in mind during aftercare appointments.

Staining

Apart from hypoxia, staining (or even the occasional infiltrate) may be caused by entrapment of debris and reduced tear exchange, given that the lenses are designed to resist rotation.

5
Soft contact lenses in presbyopia

Introduction   70
Presbyopia   71
Soft contact lenses in presbyopia   73
Monovision   74
   Partial monovision   76
   Enhanced monovision   76
   Modified monovision   77
Soft multifocal lenses and pupil size   77
Center-near aspheric lenses   78
Distance center multizonal lenses   79
Modified monovision   80
Diffractive bifocal lenses   81
References   81

Introduction

In the developed world, we are told that the population is aging. In 1991, 37.1% of the UK population was over 45 years of age, and it is projected that by 2011 this figure will have risen to 43.5%. The average age of the population increased from 34.1 years in 1971 to 38.2 years in 2002, and is expected to rise to 43.3 years by 2031. Individuals live longer, and the birth rate is falling. The number of people requiring optical correction of their presbyopia is also therefore increasing. Realistically, the 45–65 year group is probably the target market for multifocal contact lenses, and most of the first-time users of multifocal lenses will be at the lower end of the age range. The early presbyope often has more disposable income than at any other time in their life. The children are in higher education or gainful employment, the mortgage has been paid off, and the career is peaking. To avoid the use of reading glasses, many will consider multifocal contact lenses, if they are given the slightest encouragement by their eye care professionals. They consist both of current contact lens wearers and those who are purely spectacle wearers, although the latter group will contain some individuals who have worn lenses in the past. The onset of presbyopia used to be one of the events that precipitated drop-out from contact lens wear, due to the lack of a viable multifocal option at the time, and there are some previous wearers who would like to try contact lenses again.

In many ways, it is fortunate that it is the early presbyope who usually wants contact lenses, as age brings other changes. Changes in the tear film, conjunctival folds and slackening of the eyelids can all complicate contact lens fitting, and the presbyopic patient is far more likely to be on long-term medication, much of which, like β-blockers and hormone replacement therapy, can contribute to dry eye. On the other hand, some long-term contact lens wearers may bear the evidence of their misspent youth, which may influence the choice of multifocal lens by the practitioner.

The ideal candidate for any form of soft lens correction for presbyopia is prepared to accept some visual compromise, especially at near distances. These lenses work well for undemanding near tasks, such as reading a menu, but tend to be less successful with critical vision tasks. They also struggle to provide higher reading additions. If patients read a lot, however, a rigid gas permeable (RGP) multifocal might be more promising. On the other hand, soft multifocal lenses are not gaze dependent, as they do not rely on lens translation, so they are useful for those who need a presbyopic correction in a range of directions of gaze. Mechanics, electricians and librarians may find this useful. However, they will probably all only find it useful if they have only a small astigmatic component to their refractive error. Anything over 0.75D usually rules out most presbyopic soft lenses. There are toric multifocal lenses available, but for the most part these have been lenses with indifferent oxygen transmission and infrequent replacement intervals. However, the SAM MF (Ultra Vision CLPL) can be supplied as a monthly replacement lens, and its 58% water content gives it respectable oxygen transmission. Much higher transmission values are likely to appear in the future.

Presbyopia

Presbyopia is an age-related progressive loss of accommodative amplitude. In 1909, Helmholtz described accommodation as occurring when contraction of the ciliary muscle releases tension in the zonular fibers. In the young eye, the elasticity of the lens and capsule allows the lens to become more spherical, and the increased curvature of the surfaces provides extra positive power. When the ciliary muscle relaxes, the elasticity of the zonular fibers and the choroid pull it back into its resting state, This reintroduces tension on the zonular fibers at the edge of the lens, causing the lens to flatten. This model, although challenged, has largely been confirmed by imaging techniques. There have been two main schools of thought on the cause of presbyopia. Lenticular theories concentrate on age-related changes to the lens substance, capsule and zonular fibers. Extralenticular theories consider changes to the ciliary muscle, connective tissue and choroid. A multifactorial approach is now becoming popular, incorporating both lenticular and extralenticular elements. To a certain extent, the precise mechanism is not as important to the contact lens practitioner as it is to those involved in the development of presbyopic refractive surgery.

The onset of the processes that produce presbyopia is thought to be early in life, probably soon after the eye stops growing. Its culmination occurs around the age of 55 years, when no actual accommodation is occurring, but the age at which any individual has to bow to the inevitable depends on some other factors. Patients with small pupils have a greater depth of focus, so they may be able to focus closer at a greater age, at least in a good light. The resting pupil diameter does tend to reduce with age, but considerable variation may be produced by pathology and medication as well as ambient light conditions. Another major factor in the age of onset is height. Tall people have longer arms, and habitually hold reading material at a greater working distance. The demands of near vision vary greatly between individuals, and the patient who primarily works at a VDU and rarely reads may not be troubled for some years later than a colleague who reads novels. Even the font size of the chosen daily paper may influence the moment when we all realize that presbyopia does not just happen to other people.

Myopes with medium to high spectacle prescriptions are often rather smug when their hyperopic and emmetropic colleagues submit to presbyopia. They can exploit the power change induced by looking obliquely through the lower part of the lens. In effect, they have free reading addition long before they have to admit to needing it, and the diopter or so provided by this can be further enhanced by pulling the spectacles down the nose. This increases the back vertex distance and thus decreases the effective negative power of the spectacles. However, if such a patient decides to use contact lenses, they can receive an unpleasant shock when they attempt to read, since neither of these strategies will be available. To add to their woes, accommodative demand is greater with contact lenses than it is with a myopic spectacle correction. This should, of course, result in a greater amount of accommodative convergence becoming available to reduce their exophoria. This is just as well, as convergence demand is also increased, and the rather useful base-in prism that their spectacles used to provide has disappeared. To summarize, if we fit a myopic early presbyope with contact lenses, we may induce near-vision problems associated with both feeble accommodation and/or decompensated exophoria. The situation may be different if the myope habitually reads or uses a VDU without spectacles. In this case, correcting the myopia with contact lenses could place considerable extra demands on accommodation, and this in turn could precipitate an esophoria. Given that the negative fusional reserves appear to reduce with age, decompensation is a possibility here. In comparison, hyperopes can usually switch to contact lenses relatively easily, although they can miss the extra magnification that spectacles provide and this may be reflected in their visual acuity. They will gain in terms of visual field size, however.

When a reading addition is introduced, the accommodative demand for a given distance will be reduced, and with it the amount of accommodative convergence available. Therefore, the functional reserves must be adequate to ensure comfortable binocular vision. The incorporation of horizontal prism in a multifocal contact lens is not a viable option.

Soft contact lenses in presbyopia

For the presbyopic soft lens wearer who wishes to continue with lenses, there are a number of alternatives:

1. **Single vision contact lenses** for distance and the use of spectacles for near vision as required. This does rather defeat the original object of contact lens wear, but it is nevertheless a popular option with both practitioner and patient. It is simple, and the visual acuity obtained is usually excellent. It is also cost-effective, as many patients use ready-made spectacles to supplement their distance contact lenses. However, the binocular considerations outlined above may cause difficulties if the lenses are not properly centered for the patient.

2. **Monovision** describes the process of fitting lenses to correct one eye for distance and one eye for near vision. Studies have shown that this has higher success rates than multifocal contact lens fitting, but it does not suit everyone.

3. **Multifocal contact lenses** can be divided into two main categories, alternating vision and simultaneous vision. **Alternating vision** lenses are required to *translate*, or move relative to the pupil. The advantage of this approach is that all of the light entering the pupil area is focused for the same distance, so the vision should suffer less degradation. The disadvantage is the skill and time required to fit them well. These are almost invariably rigid gas permeable (RGP) lenses, as on the whole it is relatively easy to get an RGP lens to decenter. Attempts have been made to develop a successful soft alternating design, the most recent being the Triton Translating Bifocal (Gelflex Laboratories, Australia). However, the increased thickness of a lens of this type will impact on the oxygen transmission, and it has always been difficult to obtain adequate translation with soft lenses. Lenses in the **simultaneous vision** category are expected to stay pretty much where they are, and most soft lens multifocal designs are of this type. They are normally easier to fit, but involve more visual compromise, as a significant proportion of the light entering the pupil from the object of regard will not focus in the retinal plane. The simplest form of simultaneous lens has concentric zones of distance and near power, but mostmodern lenses have aspheric or multizonal surfaces, allowing a progressive power function analogous to a varifocal spectacle lens.

Monovision

The basic principle in monovision is to correct one eye for distance and one for near vision, and on the whole it works quite well. Estimates of the success rate vary widely between 50% and 86%, depending on the criteria used to define success, but numerous studies have consistently found monovision to be rather more successful than multifocal fitting, and it is generally a simpler process. Furthermore, conventional single vision lenses can be used, and these will usually fit better, and involve less physiologic compromise, than any multifocal lens.

The ability to suppress detrimental blur information is significantly higher in successful monovision patients, but predicting who has this ability in a clinical setting is challenging. Alternating squinters are ideal, as they are well practiced in suppression of the non-fixating eye. Strong ocular dominance may be an asset when the dominant eye is fully corrected, but could be a distraction when the other eye is the one being used. Patients who report high levels of 'ghosting' during a monovision contact lens trial may be poor candidates for monovision. Other characteristics that might indicate a more guarded prognosis include age and psychological traits. Older patients tend to be less successful, as they may be less adaptable and they need higher reading additions to see clearly. Structured, detail-oriented and pessimistic people are less successful than holistic, adaptable optimistic ones.

The question of which eye to correct for distance is also challenging. For a thorough review of the literature, see Evans (2006). Conventionally, the distance correction is applied to the 'dominant' eye, determined by a sighting test, but this does not guarantee the best visual result. Alternatively, the +2.00 test described by Michaud et al (1995) may be employed. Essentially, this consists of placing a +2.00 lens in front of each eye in turn, and comparing the distance vision. If the vision is best with the +2.00 before the left eye, then the right eye is considered the dominant eye for distance. This is fairly reliable if distance vision is a priority, but this is not always the case. The best way to establish whether monovision will work and which way round to correct the eyes is to try it. This is best done in the form of an extended trial over several days, so that the patient may experience the effect at home and in the workplace. Disposable soft lenses make this a relatively inexpensive process.

Those patients who do not adapt to monovision may experience a number of problems. Blur may be experienced by those who do not suppress it efficiently, especially at night, when glare or haloes can make night driving difficult. About a third of monovision patients report this. Stereopsis will be adversely affected, yet this rarely seems to be noticed by patients. However, it may be worth mentioning to them as a precaution against future litigation. Finally, decompensation of binocular vision is a rare complication, probably because most of the patients likely to be affected have some ability to suppress.

Partial monovision

Full correction of the near vision may be impractical. Pardhan and Gilchrist (1990) found that at a point between 1.00D and 1.50D, the eyes crossed over from binocular summation to binocular inhibition. When binocular summation is occurring, the binocular contrast sensitivity is about 40% higher than the monocular. With binocular inhibition, the binocular sensitivity is lower than the monocular. This correlates well with anecdotal evidence from contact lens practitioners and refractive surgeons that additions below +1.50 work better. However, a high addition might help to stabilize blur suppression in some cases, so there may be exceptions to the rule.

Enhanced monovision

A variation on the monovision theme is to fit one eye with a single vision lens and the other with a multifocal lens. Usually, this involves a single vision distance lens in the dominant eye and a multifocal lens in the other. The idea is to improve distance vision, usually for driving, while allowing at least casual near vision. This may be a useful option for the early presbyope, who can go over to bilateral bifocal correction later on. Other variations include a single vision near/distance-biased multifocal combination, and a slightly over-plussed single vision distance/intermediate-biased multifocal for a VDU user.

Modified monovision

This involves fitting both eyes with a multifocal lens, but biasing one eye more for distance and one eye for near. This can be achieved by adjusting the power of the lens. Under-correcting the reading addition will bias a lens towards distance vision, and over-plussing the distance correction puts the bias towards near vision. Alternatively, a different design of multifocal lens may be used in each eye. A distance center lens in one eye and a near-center lens in the other is a popular combination.

Soft multifocal lenses and pupil size

The simplest and earliest soft multifocal designs employed an optic zone divided into concentric areas of spherical power for distance and near. These could be made with the distance power in the center ('center-distance or 'CD') or the periphery ('center-near' or 'CN'). This meant that for either distance, only some of the light from the object of regard would be focused accurately on the retina and that other objects in the field of vision that were situated at the other fixation distance would also be focused. Potentially, then, visual confusion and blur could ensue, as well as loss of contrast. The patient had to suppress the unwanted images in order to see the object of regard, and the ability to do this varies from patient to patient. However, any patient will find this easier if the 'signal-to-noise ratio' is high, and this ratio is largely dependent on the pupil. A large pupil will allow light from both power zones into the eye. A small pupil will favor the central power zone over the peripheral one. Unfortunately, the pupil diameter is rather variable. Individual variation can give rise to pupils between 2 mm and 7 mm, and emotional state, health and medication can change it. About a quarter of the population have pupil diameters that are unequal between their two eyes by at least 0.5 mm. The pupils constrict with near fixation, and also with increasing ambient light levels, and this can cause problems. A CD lens will give relatively good distance vision in bright conditions, but the near vision is likely to be compromised. The CN version will give better near vision in good light, but on a bright day the distance vision may be problematic, especially when driving. With the advent of modern CNC (computer numeric controlled) lathes, contact lens manufacturers can generate sophisticated surfaces on their lenses, and a number of ingenious designs have been developed to overcome the pupil problem.

Center-near aspheric lenses

The use of aspheric surfaces has enabled manufacturers to offer multifocal lenses that have a truly progressive function similar to that of a progressive spectacle lens. Most of those available are of CN design, and a popular example is the Focus Progressive, which has daily and monthly disposable versions. This design has a nominal reading addition of +3.00, although without lens translation the effective addition is likely to be about half this value. Initial lens choice is from a bank of lenses, based on the patient's refractive error and spectacle reading addition. This can be made either from a selection table provided by the manufacturer or by applying the following formula:

$$\text{Trial lens power} = \frac{\text{Spherical equivalent of spectacle}}{\text{prescription} + (\text{reading addition}/2)}$$

For example, if the best vision sphere was −3.00DS and the reading addition required +1.50:

$$\text{Trial lens power} = -3.00 + (1.50/2) = -2.25\text{DS}$$

The lenses should be given some time to settle, and 20 minutes appears to be the most common interval. Ideally, the patient should wander about outside the consulting room to get a better idea of the effect of the lenses. After this period, provided that the fit and movement of the lens is physiologically acceptable (it is a one-fit lens), the power can be refined. A good starting point is to ask the patient to score distance and near vision out of 10. Any score over 7 tends to indicate a potentially successful outcome, and 8 or above for both distances is unlikely to be improved upon. Scores below 5 probably indicate a rethink.

Over-refraction of these lenses is best done binocularly and unfogged, and this can cause some initial anxiety among practitioners used to monocular or Humphriss-style refraction. However, it does work best for these lenses. The use of refractor heads (phoropters) and reduced-aperture trial lenses is also best avoided, as they restrict the amount of light entering the eye, and will therefore cause the pupil to dilate.

Poor distance vision may be addressed initially by offering −0.25DS binocularly, and checking whether distance vision improves. If it does, the next step is to check whether the change will compromise near vision. If near vision is unaffected, the power change may be incorporated. If near vision is compromised by a binocular change in power, the next step is to try −0.25DS before each eye in turn, checking distance and near vision at each step. It is rare that bigger changes in power will result in a better lens.

Poor near vision may be addressed in a similar way, trying first binocular, and then monocular addition of +0.25DS. Where the power changes are monocular, a form of modified monovision is being employed, and many practitioners regard this as a default strategy.

Distance center multizonal lenses

CN lenses have the drawback that on a bright day, distance vision can be poor, and in low light, near vision suffers. One approach to counter this is to incorporate a number of alternating rings of distance and near power. The Acuvue Bifocal (Johnson and Johnson) incorporates five such rings over an 8 mm optic zone whose size and placement are based on research on pupil behavior in the presbyopic population. Remember, though, that these lenses are optimized for average patients. The resulting design is described by the manufacturers as 'pupil intelligent'.

There is a choice of reading additions in 0.50 steps between +1.00DS and +2.50DS. Many practitioners habitually adopt a modified monovision approach with these lenses, reducing the addition of the 'distance eye' by 0.50–1.00DS to reduce distance blur, and to improve intermediate vision.

Modified monovision

As indicated, many practitioners favor a modified monovision approach when fitting soft multifocal lenses, either by reducing the addition of the 'distance' eye or by fitting a CN lens in one eye and a CD lens in the other. At one time, this often meant using two lenses of different design, from different manufacturers, which complicated matters somewhat, particularly for disposable lenses. Coopervision has simplified things with its Frequency 55 and Proclear Multifocal lenses, by offering matched pairs of lenses. The lenses both have central and peripheral spherical zones bridged by an aspheric intermediate zone, but one is CD and one is CN. The CD lens has a central distance zone of 2.3 mm, surrounded by a 5 mm diameter aspheric annulus and a near spherical band. The diameter of the entire optic zone is 8.5 mm. The CN lens is similar, but the central near circle has a diameter of 1.7 mm. These 'balanced progressive technology' lenses should complement each other and allow binocular summation over a range of ambient light conditions.

Once the initially selected initial lenses have settled, the process of optimizing distance and near vision is similar to that described for the Focus Progressive. With a modified monovision approach, improvement of distance vision will usually involve adding ±0.25DS to the distance prescription without changes to the reading addition. To maximize near vision, +0.25DS added to the distance power of the CN lens will often improve matters, and this should always be tried first before changing the power of the reading addition. Over-prescribing of the reading addition will usually compromise distance vision.

Diffractive bifocal lenses

These lenses had a phase plate worked on to the back surface of the lens, achieved by etching a series of facets 3 μm deep in a concentric pattern. Distance vision is conventionally corrected by refraction, but near vision is corrected by a combination of refraction and diffraction. The lenses suffer from loss of contrast similar to any simultaneous vision lens, but 20% of the light is also lost to higher-order diffraction, so low-contrast acuities tend to be poor. They are largely independent of pupil size, but dependent on lens centration. They were marketed as Echelon but, currently, they appear to have become unavailable.

References

Evans B (2006) Monovision: a systematic review. *Ophthalmic Physiol Opt* (in press).
Michaud L, Tchang JP, Baril C and Gresset J (1995) New perspectives in monovision: a study comparing aspheric with disposable lenses. *Int Contact Lens Clin* **22**: 203–208.
Pardhan S and Gilchrist J (1990) The effect of monocular defocus on binocular contrast sensitivity. *Ophthalmic Physiol Opt* **10**:33–36.

6
Extended wear and silicone hydrogels

Introduction   84
Chronic hypoxia and the cornea   85
Silicone hydrogels   86
Suitability for extended wear   89
  Blepharitis   91
  Meibomian gland dysfunction   91
  Dry eye   91
  Palpebral conjunctival changes   91
  Infiltrates and scars   92
  Neovascularization   92
  Smoking   92
  Poor compliance   93
Initial lens selection   93
Collection and aftercare   95
Solutions   97
Adverse reactions   97
References   99
Further reading   99

Introduction

It is probable that contact lenses have been worn overnight by some patients, with or without the collusion of the practitioners who fitted them, for as long as contact lenses have been in existence. Some of the early glass haptic lenses fitted in the 1880s are known to have been worn continuously for up to 2 years at a time, and many adventurous people have experimented since with both haptics and polymethyl methacrylate (PMMA) corneal lenses. Market research has repeatedly found a great public demand for overnight wear, although it is difficult to see why, as much of the extra wearing time provided by these lenses is spent unconscious. There is the freedom from the daily chore of removing and cleaning the lenses. There is also the convenience of clear vision upon waking, which for those with high prescriptions may be significant. In certain occupations, such as emergency services and the armed forces, the ability to spring into action without inserting lenses may be helpful. A cynic might also point out that the promiscuous might be able to put a face to last night's companion, if not necessarily a name. However, there is a suspicion that much of the aggressive marketing of extended wear that took place was driven by the contact lens industry trying to see off the commercial threat posed by refractive surgery.

Extended wear with soft lenses can be divided into two phases. The first really began in London with John de Carle, who developed the Permalens. By 1981, the Food and Drug Administration (FDA) had approved hydrogel extended wear for cosmetic correction in the USA, and by 1985 there were about four million Americans wearing lenses on an extended wear basis. In Europe, extended wear lenses never really caught on in the same way. This may have been because they were marketed less aggressively, and because of a more conservative approach on the part of practitioners. Initial results looked promising, but success was defined largely on the ability to continue to wear the lenses. As research became more sophisticated, hydrogel extended wear lenses began to look less promising.

It is now known that when the eyes are closed during sleep, the oxygen supply to the cornea is reduced and corneal edema is the result. The average cornea swells by some 4% during sleep, but can recover when the eye opens. About 8% of the swelling can be reversed during the day. Holden and Mertz (1984) defined the levels of oxygen and oxygen transmission required to avoid corneal edema. Unfortunately, the lenses available at the time did not meet these requirements. However, some lenses were approved on the basis that they came close to the transmission levels required to give 8% swelling.

There were frequent inflammatory reactions to deposit build-up and the residues from the necessary cleaning process after up to 30 nights of extended wear. This was at least partially resolved by the adoption of weekly disposable lenses. However, there was also growing concern at the number of corneal infections associated with extended wear, and the disposable option did not seem to improve matters. The bubble burst in 1989 with the publication of a study by Poggio and Schein. Extended wear patients were found to have an incidence of keratitis of 20.9/100 000 patients, compared to an incidence of 4.1/100 000 in patients wearing hydrogel lenses on a daily basis. Subsequent studies confirmed these findings, and the ensuing publicity destroyed both public and practitioner confidence in hydrogel lens extended wear for good. In 1989, the FDA recommended that extended wear be limited to less than 7 days and 6 nights before removal, although the US contact lens industry had already taken this step voluntarily. However, approval for up to 30 nights of continuous wear for silicone hydrogel lenses has been granted in both the USA and Europe following successful clinical trials in other countries where the regulations were not so restrictive.

Chronic hypoxia and the cornea

The development of silicone hydrogel lenses has provided a great deal of information on the effects of hypoxia on corneal integrity. The main effects are seen at the three levels that contain cells.

1. The **epithelium** will show reduced cell mitosis and cell migration, and a loss of tight junctions. The result is a thinner barrier that is more easily damaged mechanically, and will recover more slowly. This, in turn, will provide greater opportunity for microbial infection.
2. The **stroma** will initially swell due to the intake of water, because the epithelium and endothelium are less able to pump it out. A build-up of carbon dioxide (hypercapnia) leads to a fall in pH (acidosis), and this can lead in time to keratocyte death, with subsequent thinning of the stroma.
3. The **endothelium** will often show signs of distress, although it is not known to what extent endothelial function is compromised. Reductions in cell count, and variations in the apparent size and shape of the cells, may be detected with the major slit-lamp. Some of these changes may not be reversible.

In addition, bacterial adherence to corneal tissue appears to be greater in hypoxic conditions.

Silicone hydrogels

Silicone hydrogels were developed in order to overcome the challenge of chronic hypoxia by meeting the Holden–Mertz criteria. The lenses that have emerged do exceed those criteria, and clinical signs of chronic hypoxia are extremely rare in patients wearing silicone hydrogel lenses. However, a little caution is desirable. The Holden–Mertz criteria are average values, and considerable variation appears to exist between individuals. Some 2% of the population show clinically detectable signs of edema (striae, folds) after closed-eye sleep, even without a contact lens, and 5% of silicone hydrogel lens wearers show similar signs, so not everyone may be suitable for extended wear with these lenses. It should also be borne in mind that Dk/t is not a simple indicator of the oxygen levels available with different lenses. Doubling the Dk/t does not double the available oxygen. Oxygen flux values give a more meaningful idea of the oxygen transmitted per unit area of cornea. Table 6.1 is a useful reminder that

Table 6.1 **Oxygen flux estimates for closed-eye wear of various lens types. Lenses are assumed to be the minimum practical thickness for –3.00 power**

Lens type	Oxygen flux ($\mu l/cm^2/h$)
Hydrogel low water content	1.8
Hydrogel medium water content	3.2
Hydrogel high water content	4.1
RGP lens Dk 25	2.6
RGP lens Dk 50	4.4
RGP lens Dk 100	5.3
Silicone hydrogel lens Dk 110	5.6
Silicone hydrogel lens Dk 140	5.7
Silicone elastomer lens	5.8

Taken from Efron N (ed.) *Contact Lens Practice*, Butterworth-Heinemann.

high-water-content hydrogel lenses were delivering about 75% of the oxygen that a silicone hydrogel lens can, and that there is a law of diminishing returns applicable to the higher levels of Dk/t.

Two lenses emerged in rapid succession in the first wave of silicone hydrogels, Focus Night and Day (CIBA) and Purevision (Bausch & Lomb). Both had oxygen transmission that easily met the Holden–Mertz criteria, but there were some important differences between them.

The material for Focus Night and Day (Lotrafilcon A 15) is described as **biphasic**, which means that the silicone (oxygen-transmitting) and hydrogel (ion-transmitting) components are arranged side by side, running in parallel from the front to the back surface. This gives excellent fluid transmission, which important to maintain lens mobility. It has a 25% water content and an oxygen transmission (Dk/t) of 175. The surface is plasma coated, resulting in a continuous surface 25 nm thick that is permanently bonded to the lens material. Initially, this lens was available with a base curve of 8.60 mm and a total diameter of 13.80 mm, but a second base curve of 8.40 mm was introduced as a result of clinical experience. At present, a back vertex power from +6.00 to −10.00 is available.

PureVision is made from Balafilcon A III 4M, a substantially homogeneous copolymer. It has a higher water content (35%), which gives it a lower oxygen transmission (110 barrer). It is a slightly more flexible lens than Focus Night and Day. The surface is plasma oxidized, which produces hydrophilic islands on the surface surrounded by hydrophobic material. The lens is available with one base curve (8.60 mm) and a total diameter of 14.00 mm, and the power range is +6.00 to −12.00. In addition, a toric option is available in spherical powers of −0.25 to −6.00 and −0.75, −1.25 and −1.75 cylinders.

Both of the preceding lenses were developed for extended wear, but it has emerged that at least half of the silicone hydrogel lenses prescribed are used for conventional daily use, or flexible wear involving part-time extended wear. Even those patients who are wearing the lenses continuously are often doing so for a shorter period than the maximum 30 days for which they are licensed.

These considerations, along with some issues regarding comfort with silicone hydrogel lenses, due to their increased rigidity when compared to a conventional hydrogel lens, have led to a second wave of lenses. These are being marketed as daily wear lenses rather than extended wear lenses, and are undoubtedly the harbingers of an extended range of silicone hydrogel lenses that will take over the soft lens market during the next few years.

Acuvue Advance with Hydraclear (Johnson & Johnson) has a high water content (45%) for a silicone hydrogel lens. This, along with its thin design, should result in a lens that is less 'stiff' than other silicone hydrogel lenses, and this may result in greater comfort for some patients, as may its enhanced wetting. However, for silicone hydrogel lenses, water content is inversely proportional to oxygen transmission, and the Dk/t barely meets the Holden–Mertz criteria for extended wear. The lens is not surface treated, but incorporates the patented Hydraclear technology. A long-chain molecule that is a derivative of the wetting agent polyvinylpyrrolidone (PVP) is incorporated in the lens matrix. It is available in base curves of 8.30 mm and 8.70 mm and a total diameter of 14.00 mm. The power range is −6.00 to +4.00. This lens is intended to be replaced at 2-weekly intervals rather than the monthly intervals of other silicone hydrogel lenses. A toric version has also been announced.

Acuvue Oasys with Hydraclear (Johnson & Johnson) is made from senofilcon A, which is claimed to be 50% smoother than other silicone hydrogel materials, and has an improved formulation of the Hydraclear technology. The water content is 38% and the Dk/t 147, which makes it an option for extended wear. It also has a UV blocking tint.

AirOptix (CIBA) has a lower water content than Purevision and a slightly higher DK/t, so it is suitable for extended wear. However, it is currently being aimed at the daily wear market and priced to compete with conventional hydrogel monthly replacement lenses. The excellent oxygen transmission and enhanced wetting capabilities of second-generation silicone hydrogel lenses should enable them to replace hydrogel lenses as first-choice monthly disposables. However, some patients still find these lenses less comfortable than hydrogel lenses. At present, AirOptix (CIBA) is available in a range of powers from +4.00 to −10.00, but no toric lenses are as yet being produced.

Suitability for extended wear

Most patients who express an interest in extended wear have no particular motivation beyond that of convenience. However, some patients will derive extra benefit from these lenses. The ability to wear these lenses for long and irregular hours may be of use to:

1. emergency service personnel
2. parents with young children
3. carers
4. armed forces personnel.

Equally, certain patients who would have difficulty in handling a conventional lens may find extended wear a useful option:

1. those with high to moderate prescriptions; at present, these lenses are only available in a limited range
2. elderly or physically impaired patients
3. patients with sight impairment; it may be possible to arrange a Galilean telescope with a high-minus contact lens and a high-plus spectacle lens
4. young children with anisometropia.

In certain therapeutic situations, extended wear would be useful:

1. bandage lens
2. drug delivery
3. piggy-back carrier.

However, setting aside all of the above, the contact lens-wearing public like the idea of extended wear:

1. Surveys have shown that 35% of soft lens wearers do not want to insert and remove lenses daily.
2. In 1986, one-third of soft lens patients wore lenses on an extended wear basis at least some of the time.
3. In 2000, 32% of 1–2 week lens wearers said that they sleep in their lenses.

There are several factors that can increase the hazards associated with extended wear, and the patients must be made aware of any that affect them:

1. blepharitis
2. meibomian gland dysfunction (MGD)
3. dry eye
4. palpebral conjunctival changes
5. infiltrates and scars
6. neovascularization

7. smoking (in young patients)
8. poor compliance with daily lens care.

Blepharitis

The staphylococcal form of blepharitis will cause burning and itchy eyes and erythema of the lid margins. Punctate staining and peripheral infiltrates are also seen. The high levels of Gram-positive bacteria present will increase the risks of inflammation and microbial keratitis.

The seborrheic form is often associated with dry eye.

Meibomian gland dysfunction

Patients with MGD often have dry-eye symptoms, and there is a higher level of Gram-positive bacteria. The incidence of contact lens-related papillary conjunctivitis (CLPC) is also higher. Treatment may be required before any contact lens wear is advisable.

Dry eye

Many patients report symptoms of 'dry eye' with or without contact lenses, but not all actually have dry eyes. Patients with severe symptoms or staining should be avoided, but those without staining may be successful, and some find silicone hydrogel lenses more comfortable than hydrogel lenses.

Patients with 'smile stain' may be better with silicone hydrogel lenses but need careful monitoring.

Palpebral conjunctival changes

Those with an atopic history often present with upper palpebral conjunctival hyperemia and large papillae on the tarsal plate. These patients are more likely to develop CLPC, especially with 'stiffer' lenses such as silicone hydrogel lenses. They may be better off with daily disposable lenses.

Infiltrates and scars

The significance of both infiltrates and scars will depend upon the cause. If this is unknown, in general the deeper they are, the more serious the likely cause. Some patients present with one or more small superficial asymptomatic infiltrates that are probably related to environmental factors and of little consequence. However, the presence of larger or deeper opacities does suggest increased risk of inflammatory events. Peripheral sterile infiltrates have a 30% recurrence rate and may be associated with Gram-positive bacterial exotoxins. McNally (2003) reported the following increased risk factors for corneal events:

- prior history of corneal scar, 4.1×
- prior history of contact lens-associated red eye (CLARE), 6.9×
- prior history of corneal infiltrates, 5.9×.

Neovascularization

In most patients, the increased oxygen levels available with silicone hydrogel lenses will mean that any new vessels induced by previous lens wear will probably empty. However, this does not happen for every patient. In the early days of silicone hydrogel lenses, it was widely thought that hyperemia simply did not occur, but work at Aston using digital imaging techniques has disproved this.

The presence of neovascularization per se does not indicate increased risk of inflammation (McNally, 2003), although localized neovascularization may be related to inflammatory events.

Smoking

McNally found that smoking more than doubled the chances of an inflammatory event, but only in the under-30s.

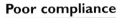
Poor compliance

Contact lens patients as a whole are not perfectly compliant with their care regimes, but those whose compliance is particularly questionable will have a rather better opportunity to damage themselves during extended wear. Patients who cannot or will not understand the risks should not be given the opportunity to learn the hard way.

Initial lens selection

The first thing to decide is whether the lenses are intended to be used for extended or daily wear, or some combination of both. If extended wear is required, a high oxygen transmission is necessary. In the early days, there was a rather limited choice. You could fit either a PureVision or a Night and Day, so most practitioners inserted one of each into the patient's eyes and saw which one was most comfortable and showed the better movement. If there was no difference, higher oxygen permeability was available with the Night and Day. The same principle is still useful today, but there is now one more lens (AirOptix) to consider, and Night and Day is available with two base curves. After experience with the lenses, most practitioners developed a preference for one lens or another, although most continued to use both Purevision and Night and Day on appropriate patients. For Purevision and AirOptix, there is only one base curve available, but for Night and Day there are two options. CIBA recommends trying the 8.40 base curve first, moving to the 8.60 option only if the 8.40 lens appears too tight. A Cornea and Contact Lens Research Unit (CCLRU) study found that the 8.60 mm base curve was successful in 74% of cases, and an alternative that is popular with practitioners is to select the 8.60 option for corneas with K values over 7.40 and only go steeper if the lenses are uncomfortable or fluting occurs.

The greater stiffness and elasticity of a silicone hydrogel lens means that a well-fitting lens should move a little more than an

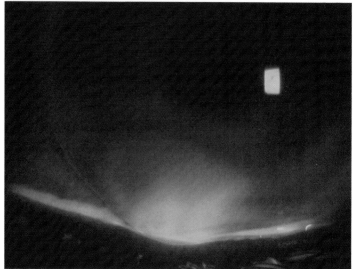

a

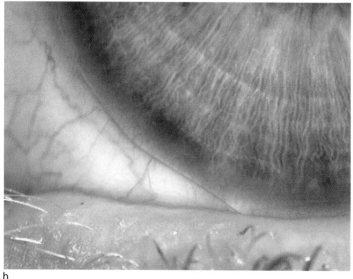

b

Figure 6.1 Fluting seen under white (a) and blue (b) light (courtesy of B. Tompkins).

equivalent hydrogel lens. Post-blink movement of 0.50–0.70 mm in both primary gaze and elevation is desirable, particularly in an extended wear lens. The push-up test should reveal a lens that feels slightly loose. High-molecular-weight fluorescein has been used to make lens 'fluting' more apparent, but most practitioners do not find this particularly useful. Fluting is a characteristic of a lens that is too loose, and may cause discomfort (Fig. 6.1).

Collection and aftercare

Before commencing overnight wear, it is important that we know that the patient can wear the lenses successfully on a daily basis. For those patients who already wear soft contact lenses, this is an easy question to answer, as the lenses that they have been wearing are likely to present rather more of a physiologic challenge than a silicone hydrogel lens will. For those new to contact lenses, a period of daily wear is needed to bring us to the same point, and this is typically 1 or 2 weeks. It is essential, therefore, that every wearer is taught to handle, clean and disinfect their lenses initially in the same way as any other soft lens wearer.

Provided that the first aftercare visit goes well, a second appointment can be made for the day following the first night of overnight wear. In theory, this examination should be conducted as soon as the patient is awake, as any signs of hypoxia will disperse rapidly, but this is obviously not possible. This appointment rarely gives rise to any important findings, but it is there as a safety net, to catch any patient who has an abnormal corneal oxygen requirement or propensity towards inflammation. Subsequent appointments at 1 week, 1 month, 3 months and then every 3–6 months should then be a minimum requirement for an uneventful patient.

The fact that these lenses are licensed for up to 30 days extended wear does not mean that they have to be worn for this long. With extended wear hydrogel lenses, longer wearing periods were associated with more infection, and although this appears to be less of a consideration with silicone hydrogel lenses, many practitioners are more comfortable with a week or so of continuous wear followed by removal and cleaning. Even better, the lenses could be worn on a daily basis with the option of overnight wear occasionally.

Extended wear patients must be educated to respond to adverse signs without delay. They should be encouraged to carry out a self-assessment of the lenses every morning by asking:

1. **Do the eyes look good?** (i.e. white – hyperemia is not a normal sign with these lenses).
2. **Do they feel good?** Are the lenses moving well? If not, an ocular lubricant may help. Lens movement is essential to flush debris from beneath the lens, and an immobile lens is likely to cause an inflammatory reaction, or worse.
3. **Can I see well?** Check each eye in turn.

If the answer to any of these questions is no, they should remove the lenses and contact their practitioner as soon as possible. Herein lies an ethical dilemma. Do you give your patients your home or mobile phone number? If you do, there is a chance that the only people who will use it will be the very individuals who you would least like to possess your personal phone numbers. If you do not, the patients must be supplied with an out-of-hours contact number, either a dedicated helpline or local hospital casualty department (it is polite to ask them first). Practice staff must be well briefed on the correct advice to give any contact lens patient who calls with a query, and if the instruction on handling and lens care is delegated, the practitioner has a responsibility to ensure that the advice given is appropriate. In particular, the patient must be told not to wear the lens if they are unwell, as there is a strong correlation with microbial keratitis. In general, a patient reporting any adverse reaction to extended wear lenses should be advised to remove them and be seen at the first opportunity, as serious complications can develop within hours.

Solutions

A certain amount of confusion surrounds the care systems for silicone hydrogel lenses. Reports of lens–solution incompatibilities began shortly after the first silicone hydrogel lenses were released. Confusion reigned, and there was a feeling that polyhexanide (polyhexamethyl biguanide, PHMB) solutions should not be used with silicone hydrogel lenses, as they caused more corneal staining than peroxide or polyquad-based systems. However, the role of polyhexanide itself had been oversimplified, and some polyhexanide-based systems cause as little staining as peroxide or polyquad-based systems. The greatest incidence of staining occurred when ReNu MultiPlus was used with Purevision lenses, but since this solution and a number of others have been reformulated, there are no reported incompatibilities between multipurpose solution care systems and any silicone hydrogel lens. Recently, Renu with Moistureloc (Bausch & Lomb) and Focus Aqua (CIBA) have been specifically targeted at silicone hydrogel lenses.

Adverse reactions

The adverse reactions seen with extended wear are in general no different from those that occur with daily wear, but their frequency and severity may be greater. A more detailed discussion of these findings is given in Chapter 9.

Common initial findings include:

1. **Lens awareness**. Silicone hydrogel lenses are stiffer and more elastic than conventional hydrogel lenses, and this may increase lid sensation. Most patients get over it, but a few never do, and refitting with a more conventional lens for daily wear may be required. Sometimes the problem can be solved by trying one of the other silicone hydrogel lenses, but the correct choice is unpredictable.

2. **Mucin balls**. These are rarely a problem in themselves, but recent research has linked them to a greater incidence of inflammatory events.

3. Established lens wearers may have some **microcysts**, and when they are refitted with silicone hydrogel lenses, the microcysts will increase in number, peaking after 2 weeks. This may take 2–3 months to resolve. This response is due to the increased availability of oxygen, so at this stage it is not a cause for concern, provided that the microcysts pre-date the present lenses.

Longer-term findings may include a hyperopic shift in refraction. This again is a rebound effect from previous soft lens wear, which may induce a slight myopic shift. The refraction should be checked for this at the second or third aftercare visit.

Subsequent complications may include the following:

1. Signs of **hypoxia** are rare but not unknown. They include:
   (a) signs of acute hypoxia: (i) striae, (ii) folds
   (b) signs of chronic hypoxia: (i) microcysts, (ii) vacuoles, (iii) neovascularization, (iv) endothelial irregularities.

2. **Mechanical complications** may include:
   (a) Superior Epithelial Arcuate Lesions (SEALs). These are a little more common with silicone hydrogel lenses, due to their mechanical properties.
   (b) CPLC. This is due to mechanical rubbing rather than being a reaction to lens deposits.

Both of these have an incidence of about 5% and may require refitting with a 'softer' lens.

3. A number of inflammatory events may be encountered, ranging from the minor to the sight-threatening. In ascending order of severity, these include:
   (a) **asymptomatic infiltrative keratitis**. This is rarely of significance.
   (b) **infiltrative keratitis**. This relatively mild response is

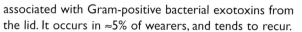
associated with Gram-positive bacterial exotoxins from the lid. It occurs in ≈5% of wearers, and tends to recur.

(c) **contact lens-associated red eye**; this can occur with extended wear. This acute reaction is associated with endotoxins from Gram-negative bacteria colonizing the lens.

(d) **contact lens peripheral ulcer**. Gram-positive bacterial toxins from organisms colonizing the lens are associated with this.

(e) **microbial keratitis**. At present, the prevalence of microbial keratitis with silicone hydrogel lenses is not entirely clear, as apparently contradictory estimates have appeared in recent publications (it would also be useful if practitioners could report diagnosed microbial keratitis events to someone who would collate data; currently, no such person/organization exists).

References

Holden BA and Mertz GW (1984) Critical oxygen levels to avoid corneal oedema for daily and extended wear. *Invest Ophthal Vis Sci* **25**: 1161–1167.

McNally JJ, Chalmers RL, McKenney CD et al. (2003) Risk factors for corneal infiltrative events with 30-night continuous wear of silicone hydrogel lenses. *Eye Contact Lens* **29**: 153–156.

Poggio EG and Schein OD (1989) The incidence of ulcerative keratitis among wearers of daily wear and extended wear soft contact lenses. *N Engl J Med* **321**: 779–783.

Further reading

Brennan NA and Chantal Coles M-L (2002) Continuous wear. In: Efron N (ed.) *Contact Lens Practice*, pp 275–293. Butterworth-Heinemann: Oxford.

Sweeney DF (2000) *Silicone Hydrogels*. Butterworth Heinemann: Oxford.

7
Collection and lens care

Introduction   102
Hygiene   102
Insertion and removal of lenses   102
Adaptation schedule   107
Recognizing normal and abnormal   108
Frequently asked questions and general advice   109
Aftercare   109
Soft lens care regimes   110
Sterilization, disinfection and cleaning   111
    Cleaning   111
    Rinsing   115
    Disinfection   115
The lens case   120
Rewetting   121
Reference   121

Introduction

The advice given at the collection (or 'teach') appointment is an important factor in the success or failure of any contact lens wear. Collection is often delegated to unqualified staff, but it remains the responsibility of the prescribing practitioner to ensure that the advice given is sound and safe.

During this appointment, the patient must be educated in the following areas:

1. the importance of hygiene
2. safe insertion and removal of their lenses
3. adaptation schedule
4. how to recognize when things are going wrong
5. the importance of regular aftercare and the probable consequences of non-compliance
6. correct use of their care regime.

Hygiene

Fingers that insert contact lenses need to have short, clean fingernails to minimize the risk to the cornea. Patients with long nails should be advised to cut them short, and the time to do this is before the lenses are fitted. Careful hand-washing is essential before handling lenses, and the practitioner should set a good example during the initial fitting process, and check during aftercare appointments that the patient has not forgotten this important step.

Insertion and removal of lenses

In order to insert a contact lens, the patient must override their own ocular defense mechanisms, and some find this easier than others. In general, females find this a little easier, provided that they have experience in applying eye make-up, but there are

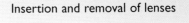
exceptions. In some cases, a dry run, without lenses, may help to overcome any squeamishness.

The lens should always be inspected before insertion to ensure that it is not damaged and that there is no debris attached. We also need to ensure that the lens is not inside out. There are several methods to ensure this:

1. Some manufacturers put small markers on their lenses. These consist of patterns or sequences of letters that will only give the correct appearance when the lens is the right way round.

2. The lens is placed on the tip of a finger and observed from the side. If it is the correct way round, it will adopt a hemispherical 'bowl' shape. If it is inverted, the edges of the lens will flare out (see Figs 3.2 and 3.3).

3. The lens is allowed to dry slightly, and then squeezed gently between finger and thumb, as if to fold it in half. If the lens is the right way round, the edges will turn inwards. An inverted lens will resist the folding, and the edges will attempt to fold back on the fingers.

4. If you are still not sure, insert the lens. If it is the wrong way round, it will be a little uncomfortable, the vision will be variable, and the lens will move excessively, rather as in the case of a loose fit. Even after insertion, it may be difficult to tell with some lenses. A patient of mine established some sort of record by never arriving for aftercare with either lens the right way round. It never seemed to cause any problems though.

The main challenge when inserting a soft lens is the size of the lens relative to the palpebral aperture. Rigid gas permeable (RGP) lenses are generally less than a centimeter in diameter, but soft lenses are half as big again, and somewhat floppy as well. It is essential, therefore, that the patient controls their eyelid and head position throughout the insertion process, and looking at their own eye in a conveniently placed mirror will help considerably, at least at first. To insert the right lens, the lens is placed on the tip of either the first or middle finger of the right hand (to insert the right lens), depending on patient preference. It helps if the applying fingertip is as dry as possible before placing the lens ('dry finger, wet lens'), and dabbing it on a lint-free tissue before picking up the lens may help the lens to transfer to the eye.

The patient is instructed to look down. The left hand is brought to rest on the forehead, and the tip of the middle finger is placed on the upper lid margin of the right eye, inside the lashes. The lid is pulled up, and provided that the placement of the finger is correct, the patient should be unable to blink with the finger in place. The patient is then instructed to look into the mirror. The lower lid is gently pulled down by the tip of either the middle or ring finger of the right hand, depending on which feels more comfortable to the patient. The lens is then applied to the cornea, with the patient encouraged to maintain fixation on their eye in the mirror, so as to counteract Bell's phenomenon. Alternatively, the lens may be applied to the upper or lower sclera. To target the lower sclera, the patient lowers their chin and looks upwards. This method has the advantage that it is a little less likely to trap debris under the optic zone. Once the lens is on the sclera, a few good blinks should center it on the cornea, but if this is not the case, the lens can be slid into place with a finger or using the lower lid. Once the lens is thought to be on the cornea, the patient should check that they can see with the lens.

New wearers tend to approach the eye with the lens extremely slowly, which gives them far more opportunity to lose their nerve, and the lens more scope to dry. They also have a tendency to let go of the lids and look away from the mirror at the moment of insertion. Gentle coaching is required to overcome this, and patience is required.

Removal of a soft lens is generally easier than insertion. Three methods are commonly employed:

1. The eyelids are held in exactly the same way as for insertion, and the lens is gently pinched off between a finger and the thumb. Ideally, the lens should be moved off the cornea first. This can be achieved by placing a finger on the lens and sliding it down onto the lower sclera. Patients who omit this step may present at aftercare appointments with lower corneal

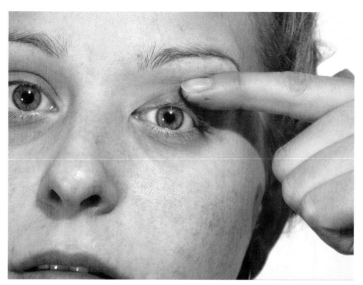

Figure 7.1 Removal of lenses must be checked at aftercare appointments

staining, which may mimic that associated with drying. For any patient who exhibits lower corneal staining, particularly in the 4 and 8 o'clock positions, it is worth checking how they remove their lenses (Fig. 7.1).

2. Some patients find it easier to slide the lens temporally. When it reaches the outer canthus, it will usually fold and pop out. Unfortunately, it sometimes does so in a direction that is not entirely predictable, and the lens may be lost. This is probably the safest method for someone with long fingernails. However, cutting the nails would be preferable (Fig. 7.2).

3. The lens can be removed by pinching it between the upper and lower lid margins, which are each controlled by a finger (Fig. 7.3). This works best if it has some stiffness, so it is more appropriate for a silicone hydrogel lens than it would be for a daily disposable lens. A wide palpebral aperture is also a prerequisite, in view of the large diameter of most soft lenses.

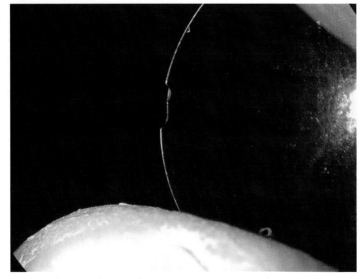

Figure 7.2 Lens damage from long nails is common (courtesy of D. Ruston)

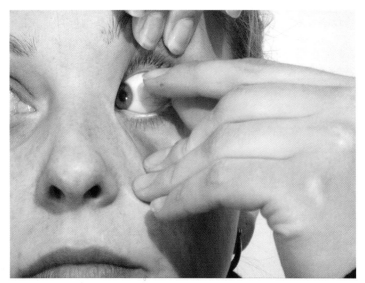

Figure 7.3 'Pinching' works with higher-modulus lenses

Whatever method is used, new patients should be seen to insert and remove their lenses at least three times. Established wearers should be observed at least once to ensure that their technique is safe. Occasionally, they may need to be re-educated, particularly if they are damaging a lot of lenses.

Adaptation schedule

There is not a lot to adapt to with a modern lens. Soft lenses are usually comfortable soon after first insertion, although those with thicker edges (e.g. torics) or a stiffer constitution (e.g. silicone hydrogels) may take a little longer. All lenses will restrict the oxygen supply somewhat, but less than the older designs used to do. However, it is customary to build up wearing time gradually, as an unsatisfactory lens will have less opportunity to cause problems before it is noticed. Typically, the patient is instructed to wear the lens for 4 hours on the first day, and add an extra 2 hours a day subsequently. In general, wear is restricted to 8 hours maximum until the first aftercare appointment. Once the fit is deemed to be optimal, there seems little point in setting a maximum wearing time, provided that it is understood that overnight wear is inappropriate for lenses intended for daily wear. If wearing time needs to be restricted beyond this, you need to fit a better lens. Patients rarely take much notice of arbitrary maxima for wearing their lenses, and if they exceed them without any consequences, the credibility of the practitioner will be compromised. A 10 hour maximum wearing time enthusiastically recommended by many optometry students is especially foolish, as the average working member of the population is likely to be traveling home, and the authors do not recommend either removing or inserting contact lenses while on the move. Restrictions on wearing time should be based on clinical findings suggestive of physiologic compromise, not picked at random.

Provided that the instruction on handling has not left the patient with too much trauma (and it is wise to check), it will boost confidence if the patient can leave the practice wearing the lenses.

Recognizing normal and abnormal

It is important that the patient should be able to tell the difference between the normal symptoms that accompany adaptation to lenses and those circumstances that require intervention. In general, soft lenses are comfortable more or less immediately, and should remain so. Mild foreign body sensation may be expected with some toric, multifocal and silicone hydrogel lenses, but it should soon decrease. Some lens awareness may be anticipated as the lens dries during prolonged wear. Significant redness and/or discomfort, especially if persistent after lens removal, should be recognized as abnormal. The patient should be advised to suspend lens wear and contact the practitioner promptly. Reduction in vision should elicit a similar response, although it might be worth checking whether the lenses are in the correct eyes before taking further action. Most patients have managed to mix up their lenses at some time, and one of the authors once managed to drive to work with both lenses in the same eye.

The Opticians Act 1989 (Amendment) Order obliges the last practitioner to participate in the fitting of the lenses to provide:

1. a signed, written specification of the lenses fitted
2. instructions and information on the care, wear, treatment, cleaning and maintenance of the lens.

The specification should be issued once you are satisfied with the lens. This would normally be after the first aftercare appointment. The instructions on lens care must be issued at the time of collection.

Patients need to be aware of the possible consequences of poor lens care, and should have the opportunity to ask questions. It is worth reinforcing verbal instructions with written information, as much of the former may be forgotten. Most practitioners issue a standard consent form, which is signed by the patient (or guardian in the case of a minor) to acknowledge that the proper advice and instructions have been given. A copy should be kept with the clinical records, and one issued to the

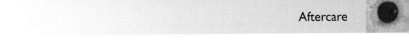

patient. The exact legal status of such declarations has never been tested in a UK court, but it is better than nothing.

Frequently asked questions and general advice

Some common questions may arise upon collection of the lenses, or at subsequent appointments:

1. **If I don't wear these lenses every day, can I replace them less frequently than a month?** The answer to this is no, as the lenses are only licensed for 30 days from the opening of the package. However, many patients do wear monthly lenses for longer (and daily ones too). Both the lenses and their care systems are not designed for more prolonged lifespans, and the risk of both increased lens deposits (leading to inflammatory reactions) and microbial keratitis will increase.

2. **Can I swim in them?** Opinions vary on this, but there is an increased risk of microbial keratitis associated with both swimming and the wearing of lenses in hot tubs. For swimming, the risk is slight if goggles are worn and the lenses are discarded immediately afterwards, but in general, prescription swimming goggles are a better option.

Patients should also be advised that tap water should not come into contact with the lenses, because of the increased risk of *Acanthamoeba* infection. They should also never wear their lenses when unwell, as there is an increased risk of microbial keratitis. Smokers (at least those under 30 years of age) are also known to be more likely to develop microbial keratitis, but I have never encountered one who gave up the habit for this reason.

Aftercare

The new regulations place the practitioner under a duty to 'make arrangements' for the wearer to receive aftercare, without actually defining aftercare. This obligation applies in circumstances and over a time period that is reasonable in a particular case, but the patient should not leave the practice with lenses unless an aftercare schedule has been discussed, and the first appointment preferably booked. It is customary to see the patient 1–2 weeks after collection, but individual patients may require other intervals.

Soft lens care regimes

The care of soft contact lenses used to be an involved and time-consuming process. Each step of the process required a separate solution or tablet that had to be diluted in another solution. Not surprisingly, patient compliance with these complex systems was indifferent, sometimes with unfortunate consequences. In particular, omission of surface cleaning was linked to an increased incidence of microbial keratitis. Initially, the choice was between systems based on heat disinfection and systems based on chemical disinfection. Both required separate cleaning solutions and frequently the use of enzyme-containing tablets to supplement them. The emergence of systems based on hydrogen peroxide overcame many of the problems associated with previous methods, but the systems remained somewhat complex. The trend in recent years has been towards 'multipurpose' solutions. These can be used for both cleaning and storage. Their popularity has coincided with the emergence of frequent replacement lenses, and they are formulated to work with modern lens materials and modalities. At present, these solutions are undergoing rapid evolution in terms of antimicrobial efficiency and cleaning performance, as large manufacturers with large research and development budgets (and, it seems, even larger marketing budgets) compete for a market that has been curtailed by the widespread use of disposable lenses, which require no solutions.

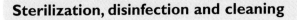

Sterilization, disinfection and cleaning

It is important to differentiate sterilization, disinfection and cleaning. Optometry students frequently employ the terms inappropriately and interchangeably.

Sterilization involves the elimination of all living microorganisms, including bacterial spores and *Acanthamoeba* cysts. This is achieved during the manufacture of lenses by the application of heat in an autoclave, typically 115–118°C for 30 minutes. When lenses arrive from the manufacturer, they will be sterile. Once the lens vial is opened, they will no longer be sterile.

Disinfection eliminates microorganisms, but bacterial spores may survive. If lenses are not disinfected, microbial keratitis is more likely to occur. Brennan and Coles (1997) found that contact lens wearers are 60 times more likely to develop microbial keratitis than are non-wearers. There are several reasons for this. Contact lenses do interfere with the ocular defense mechanisms. They prevent the efficient flushing of microorganisms and organic debris form the ocular surface, and may reduce the level of fibronectin, which may enable bacteria to adhere more easily to the cornea. However, an important factor is the increased microbial population that accompanies lens insertion.

Cleaning and **rinsing** of contact lenses removes surface deposits and debris from the lens surface. It contributes greatly to the elimination of microorganisms, and probably accounts for 99% of the disinfection process if carried out efficiently. Given the degree of compliance of the average contact lens patient, cleaning alone cannot be relied on to ensure safe wear.

Cleaning

Traditionally, separate cleaning solutions were employed, and some are still used. They are required with most peroxide-based systems, and may be required to supplement the cleaning action of multipurpose solutions. For anything up to monthly replacement, this is rarely necessary, but some patients have a tendency to deposit more than others. For lenses replaced at greater intervals, multipurpose solutions will often have inadequate cleaning potential, and a separate cleaning solution, possibly supplemented with an enzymatic cleaner at intervals, will be required in most cases.

Cleaning solutions may contain a number of cleaning agents with different modes of action.

Surfactants

Surfactants work in the same way as the detergents used to clean crockery and clothes. They dissolve debris and form a monolayer around lipid droplets; this prevents recombination and allows the lipid to be emulsified. Common surfactants include poloxamine and amphoteric imadazoline derivatives. The surfactant cleaner may be supplemented with other cleaning agents:

1. Miraflow (CIBA) contains isopropyl alcohol, which acts as a **lipid solvent**, and also has a preservative action.
2. Optifree Daily Cleaner (Alcon) has fine **polymeric beads** that have a mild abrasive action.
3. EDTA (ethylene diamine tetra-acetic acid) or one of its salts is a **chelating agent** that removes calcium ions. Calcium can act as a bridge between the lens surface and protein deposits. EDTA also has some antimicrobial action, as calcium is needed for cell wall metabolism.

Some cleaners will also contain preservatives, and buffering agents to maintain pH.

Protein removal systems

Protein removal systems are used to remove bound proteins from the lens surface. However, they need to be used before the protein becomes denatured, so occasional use is generally ineffective. For effective cleaning, weekly use is recommended. The active ingredients in these systems are enzymes:

1. **Papain** is extracted from papaya. It was the first to be employed, and can be found in Hydracare Fizzy tablets (AMO). It is an effective protein remover and is more effective than pancreatin against heavy protein deposits. However, it is associated with more ocular discomfort than more recently introduced enzymes, and adverse reactions have been reported with high-water-content lenses. For this reason, shorter soaking times are advocated with these lenses. The enzyme is neutralized by rinsing or by heat disinfection.

2. **Pancreatin** is sourced from the pancreas of pigs and oxen. It is found in Opti-free Supraclens solution (Alcon), which can be added to Opti-free Express multipurpose solution or its rigid lens equivalent for simultaneous cleaning and disinfection. Pancreatin has some action against lipid and mucoid deposits, as it contains both a lipase and an amylase in addition to the protease.

3. **Subtilisin A** is produced by controlled fermentation of bacteria (*Bacillus lichenformis*). It is less likely than papain to cause adverse reactions. Tablets containing this enzyme can be formulated so that they can be dissolved in hydrogen peroxide or in multipurpose solution. Both Ultrazyme Universal Intensive Protein Cleaner (AMO) and Unizyme (CIBA) contain this enzyme.

Multipurpose solutions

Multipurpose solutions incorporate cleaning agents that enable them to be used for both storage and cleaning. Initially, these were similar to those used in separate cleaning solutions, albeit at lower concentration, and they were designed to be used with manual 'rub-and-rinse' cleaning. This step was particularly important with early multipurpose solutions, as they were ineffective against *Acanthamoeba*. Recently developed solutions have enhanced antimicrobial and cleaning properties, which have enabled manufacturers to offer 'no-rub' formulations that eliminate this step. Practitioners are as yet not entirely convinced that this is a good thing, given the proven effectiveness of rub-and-rinse cleaning, but manual cleaning is only effective if it is done properly. Many patients were rather half-hearted in their approach to rubbing and rinsing, and some simply did not bother.

The first 'no-rub' solution available was Opti-free Express (Alcon). In addition to a poloxamine surfactant and the chelating agent EDTA, it contains a citrate buffer that has a negative charge. This attracts positively charged proteins such as lysozyme, thus reducing lens deposition. The citrate buffer is used with a polyquad (polidronium chloride) preservative.

Several other 'no-rub' solutions are now available, including ReNu MultiPlus (Bausch & Lomb), Complete (AMO), and Solocare (CIBA). These all contain polyhexanide (PHMB, polyhexamethyl biguanide) as the preservative, and borate or phosphate buffers, which reduce the tendency of this preservative to bind to the lens. It has been suggested that solutions containing polyhexanide are more likely to cause corneal staining with hydrogel and silicone hydrogel lenses, but recent research has indicated that the other components of the solution may be factors here, as solutions with similar polyhexanide concentrations appear to vary in the degree of staining caused.

Recently released solutions contain agents designed to improve the wetting of the lens surface and reduce the deposition of certain proteins. Renu with Moistureloc (Bausch & Lomb) contains two synergistic polymers. Polyquarternium 10 binds to both anionic (as in the group IV materials commonly used for frequent replacement) and non-ionic surfaces. Poloxamer 407 forms a protective shield, binding to Polyquarternium 10 and to surface debris with its hydrophobic center while attracting moisture with its hydrophilic ends. The effect is to stabilize proteins, notably tear lysozyme. In its native form, lysozyme is transparent and appears not to be associated with a reduction in lens comfort. It also has antimicrobial properties. Once it becomes denatured, it forms a visible deposit on the lens. The wettability of the lens surface is reduced, as is lens comfort, and immunologic reactions may occur. The polymers in this solution stabilize the lysozyme in its native state, and discourage deposition. Bacterial adhesion to the lens is also reduced.

Rinsing

Most rinsing these days is done using the same multipurpose solution that is used for everything else, but saline solutions are also available for use as appropriate. In earlier times, it was common to make up saline solution using tablets and (hopefully) distilled water, but home-made solutions have been associated with microbial keratitis, and tablets are no longer available for the production of saline for contact lens use. However, similar tablets are available from the home brewing sector in many outlets, and there are still patients who use these. Saline is currently available in aerosol, unit dose and multi-dose squeezy-bottle forms.

Aerosol containers resist contamination through the pressure within them, but contamination of the spray tip is not unknown, and it is a good idea to expel a small amount of saline before applying any to the lens. **Unit dose** containers share the virtue of being preservative-free, and are less bulky. This makes them particularly useful for use when traveling.

Squeezy bottles will always contain some preservative to prevent contamination. Purite saline (AMO) contains chlorine dioxide, Bausch & Lomb saline has sorbic acid, and CIBA Vision saline has a low concentration of hydrogen peroxide.

Disinfection

There are many ways to disinfect a contact lens, and most of them have been tried at some point.

Heat disinfection was a popular method in the early days of soft lenses, and it was the first method approved by the Food and Drug Administration (FDA) in the USA. A minimum of 10 minutes at 80°C is required, and most commercially available units exceed this comfortably. Heat is very effective against all of the microbes relevant to contact lens wear, including *Acanthamoeba*. Once the unit is purchased, there is little further outlay needed, but it does require a source of electricity. A more significant drawback is the effect of heat on protein, which should be familiar to anyone who has ever fried an egg. Denatured protein on the lens will reduce acuity, alter the physical parameters of the lens, and cause inflammatory reactions such as papillary conjunctivitis. When heat units were popular in the mid-1970s, the lens materials in use were often low water content and non-ionic, so protein deposition was not a major problem. However, the group IV materials in common use today have a greater affinity for protein, and a single heat cycle after a day of wear can deform and discolor such a lens. A further disadvantage of this system is that once the heat cycle is complete, the lenses are sitting in unpreserved saline, which has no antimicrobial properties. Recontamination would be rapid unless the case was completely airtight, and daily repetition of the heat cycle was essential even when the lenses were not worn. Several other methods involving radiation and sound waves have been tried:

1. **Microwave irradiation** in a domestic microwave oven is effective, but only if a microwave oven is available. Small but insignificant parameter changes have been reported.
2. **Ultraviolet** units were a common sight in practice in the 1970s. The results obtained experimentally have been mixed, particularly with respect to *Acanthamoeba*. The Purilens (American Vision) system uses UV to disinfect, in combination with subsonic turbulence for cleaning.
3. **Ultrasound** has a limited antimicrobial effect, but the similarity between the lens material and the solution requires that rather a lot of energy must be put in, and surface damage is possible.

For many years, **chemical disinfection** was achieved with solutions containing chlorhexidine gluconate or thiomersal, or a combination of both. The antimicrobial action was good, but both are smallish molecules that could penetrate into the matrix of a soft lens. Over time, they tended to concentrate and then leach out onto the ocular surface, and solution sensitivity became a common feature of soft lens wear, probably contributing to the continuing popularity of RGP lenses in this period. There was a rather novel product called OptimEyes, which consisted of a tablet which, when dissolved in tap water, became a solution containing chlorhexidine. It was cheap and effective, even against *Acanthamoeba*, but unfortunately was not suitable for group IV lenses, as chlorhexidine is less effective with ionic materials. The other slight problem was the need for rising mains tap water. Tap water became rather unpopular after the first *Acanthamoeba* scare, and this probably ensured that OptimEyes never really took off.

Chlorine-releasing agents became popular in the late 1980s and early 1990s, and about a quarter of all soft lens patients were using this method. However, by 2000 their popularity had plummeted, after research indicated an increased risk of microbial keratitis with these systems. (This may be partly attributable to the fact that the tablets were dissolved in saline. Many patients who ran out of tablets continued to carry on with saline alone, and for a while had no adverse effects.) In particular, there was a 15× greater risk of *Acanthamoeba* keratitis with chlorine systems compared to hydrogen peroxide.

Hydrogen peroxide is a highly effective antimicrobial agent. When the molecule decomposes, it produces a highly reactive hydroxyl free radical that attacks lipids and proteins within microbial cells. Three percent peroxide will kill *Acanthamoeba* trophozoites in 3 minutes and the more resistant cysts in 9 hours. It breaks down to water and oxygen, so it is environmentally friendly. Peroxide systems can also claim to be 'preservative-free', as they do not contain the chemical preservatives that cause solution sensitivity. Peroxide has long been regarded as the 'gold standard' in soft lens care. However, it does have its own drawbacks. Hydrogen peroxide needs a stabilizer to counteract its natural tendency to decompose, and one of the chemicals used, stannate, has been associated with hazing of ionic lenses. It is also toxic to the eye, and requires neutralization before the lens can be worn. Initially, this was done by immersing the lens in a separate neutralizing solution before lens insertion. In the case of Oxysept (AMO), the neutralizing solution contains the enzyme 'catalase', which neutralizes the peroxide in about a minute. Sodium pyruvate is the neutralizing agent used in 10-10 (CIBA). This achieves neutralization in about 6 minutes. Originally, the idea was to store the lens overnight in peroxide and neutralize the following morning, but many patients preferred a shorter disinfection period (10 minutes or so) before neutralizing their lenses.

Two-step systems such as Oxysept and 10-10 are complex, especially as the lenses need to be cleaned and rinsed before disinfection, and manufacturers released simpler systems that eliminated the separate neutralization phase. In the Oxysept 1-step system, the case is filled with peroxide and a tablet is added. The coating of the tablet is dissolved by the peroxide, releasing the catalase encapsulated within, which neutralizes the peroxide in about 2 hours. An alternative approach is to incorporate a platinum disk into the lens case. This acts as a catalyst, which neutralizes the peroxide over a period of about 6 hours. However, the initial reduction in concentration is extremely rapid. In the first 2 minutes, it goes from 30 000 to 9000 p.p.m. The platinum disk should be replaced every 3 months or 90 uses, but many patients are rather forgetful. This is not an entirely bad thing from the disinfection point of view, as the neutralization of the peroxide is slowed, but residual peroxide can cause irritation and discomfort.

One-step systems are popular with patients because of their convenience, but less so with practitioners. There is concern that the relatively short exposure to a high concentration of hydrogen peroxide may limit their effectiveness against *Acanthamoeba*. Although there is no statistical evidence for an increased risk of *Acanthamoeba* infection with one-step systems, there have been a few reports of apparently compliant users with *Acanthamoeba* keratitis. It should also be borne in mind that once the peroxide is neutralized, all peroxide systems lose their antimicrobial action, and re-infection may be rapid. For this reason, lenses worn infrequently should not be stored in neutralized peroxide, which is effectively saline solution.

Hydrogen peroxide does reduce lens hydration, and this in turn causes changes in total diameter and base curve, albeit temporary. After 20 minutes in the neutralizing solution, lenses

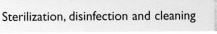
return to their original parameters. The parameter changes appear to be most marked in group IV materials, which are commonly used in frequent replacement modalities.

Multipurpose solutions now dominate the soft lens care market, with some 80% of wearers using them. They have replaced the traditional antimicrobial agents with alternatives that are less toxic to the eye. These are much larger molecules than their predecessors, which prevents penetration into the lens matrix. The most common antimicrobial used is polyhexanide, a chemical relative of chlorhexidene. Rather confusingly, it goes under a range of aliases, including dymed and polyhexamethyl biguanide. It has been used in presurgical antimicrobial scrubs and to sanitize swimming pools.

The concentration used varies from 0.6 to 5 p.p.m., with the higher concentrations providing more effective antimicrobial action but a greater potential for causing corneal staining. Group II lenses, which have an affinity for lipid to which polyhexanide can bind, have been particularly associated with this. However, it has recently become apparent that other components in the solution may be important, as solutions with the same concentration of polyhexanide have been found to give different levels of staining when used with silicone hydrogel lenses.

Polyquad is a related molecule of even higher molecular weight, and it is used in Alcon products such as Opti-free and Opti-free Express. In the latter case, a second antimicrobial agent has been added. Myristamidopropyl dimethylamine (known usually as MAPD, for obvious reasons) is included to provide effectiveness against *Acanthamoeba*, because both polyquad and polyhexanide are ineffective against it. It is claimed by the manufacturer (and disputed by some of their rivals) that this combination is as effective against *Acanthamoeba* as peroxide. There is some question about whether either is as effective against some strains of *Acanthamoeba* as they are against those used in laboratory tests. The enhanced antimicrobial ability of Opti-free Express, along with improvements to its active cleaning ability, enabled it to become the first 'no-rub' solution on the market, although others have since followed.

Alexidine is another member of the polyhexanide family, with greater effectiveness and lower toxicity. It is used in Renu with MoistureLoc, which also has polymers incorporated to enhance its cleaning action (see above).

Regard (Advanced Eye Research) has a novel antimicrobial system. **Sodium chlorite** releases chlorine dioxide in the presence of bacteria, and then reconverts to a stable solution in the case. Once outside the case, it will break down into salt water and oxygen. Regard also contains a low (100 p.p.m.) concentration of hydrogen peroxide, which acts synergistically with the sodium chlorite. At this concentration, toxic reactions would not be expected.

The lens case

The case in which the lens is stored is known to be an important potential source of infection. About three-quarters of all lens cases are contaminated with bacteria, and sometimes these include *Pseudomonas* and *Serratia*. Additionally, 8% may have *Acanthamoeba* contamination. At one time, patients used to hang on to their cases for as long as their lenses, i.e. years. By the time the case was retired, both it and the lenses it contained were often heavily deposited and probably a health hazard, since patients rarely if ever cleaned them. In time, the plastic from which the cases were constructed broke down, and some of the components released into the solution adversely affected its performance.

Some of these problems were addressed when manufacturers began to package new cases with their multipurpose solutions, but even now the human capacity for self-destructive behavior can be a formidable adversary. For some reason, patients hang on to their old case like a favorite old jumper, even when they have a new one available.

Recently, CIBA Vision released the MicroBlock lens case (Fig. 7.4), which is used with their Focus Aqua multipurpose solution. This is made from polypropylene and incorporates the

Figure 7.4 MicroBlock antibacterial lens case

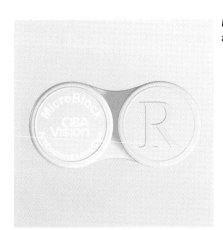

inorganic antimicrobial silver. An antimicrobial lens case may be particularly effective against those bacteria that form biofilms.

Rewetting

Contact lens patients often complain of symptoms of dryness, although research has shown that dryness may not always be the cause of those symptoms. Rewetting drops ('comfort drops') are commonly used to try to alleviate these symptoms, and they are generally found by patients to improve comfort. However, the exact mechanism is obscure, as they do not appear to improve the pre-lens tear film significantly, and the effect is probably not much greater than that of instilling saline. Some are available as single-dose, unpreserved solutions, but most contain similar preservatives to other soft lens care solutions.

Reference

Brennan NA and Coles M-LC (1997) Extended wear in perspective. *Optom Vis Sci* **74**: 609–623.

8
Aftercare

Introduction   124
Symptoms and history   124
Vision and over-refraction   127
Assessment of the lenses   128
Management of complications   129
Promoting compliance   129
References   133
Further reading   133

Introduction

The purpose of aftercare is to ensure the continued wellbeing of the patient, and the practitioner has both reactive and proactive roles. The reactive element involves gathering information from talking with the patient and clinical observation of the lenses and eyes, and then initiating appropriate management strategies. The proactive element is the encouragement of compliance with lens care that would otherwise deteriorate over time. This second goal is often pursued rather less assiduously than the first, yet it may have a profound influence on the outcome of contact lens wear. To put it another way, prevention is better than cure.

Initially, aftercare appointments could be regarded as part of the fitting process, where minor adjustments are made to the lenses or care system. Once this sequence is complete, the emphasis shifts to the longer-term consequences of lens wear, and to keeping the patient both compliant and aware of any developments in lens design or care systems that may be of benefit to them.

Symptoms and history

The first question that should be asked of any patient presenting for aftercare is: 'Are you having any problems, or is this just a routine check?'

If problems are being experienced, they are likely to concern discomfort, poor vision, or poor cosmetic appearance. For any of these, detail is important, and this should always include the following:

1. Which eye?
2. When did it first start?
3. When does it happen?
4. What seems to set it off?
5. What seems to improve it?
6. Is it getting better or worse?

Discomfort may manifest itself in several ways:

1. If it is felt immediately on insertion, it may indicate a sharp or damaged lens edge, or a reaction to solutions.
2. If it gradually gets worse over the wearing period, look for evidence of drying and deposition.
3. Pain, as opposed to discomfort, may indicate corneal damage or infection.
4. If the pain gets worse on removal, suspect corneal insult or infection.
5. Photophobia may indicate edema or inflammation.

Poor vision may also appear in several guises:

1. If it is constant, the chances are that the lens power is wrong.
2. If it is poor in one eye only, check that the lenses are in the correct eyes. Most wearers have mixed up their lenses at some point.
3. If it is transient or intermittent, drying of the lens surface, possibly secondary to lens deposits or a poor tear film, are indicated.
4. Vision that gets progressively worse throughout the wearing period may be due to edema or deposits.

The cause of **redness of the eyes** may be indicated by its distribution:

1. If it is generalized, a solution reaction should be suspected.
2. Drying may cause a band of injected vessels to traverse the bulbar conjunctiva from the inner to outer canthus.
3. Swollen eyelids and ptosis may be caused by irritation from the lens edge.
4. Perilimbal redness may be associated with hypoxia, solution sensitivity or corneal inflammation, including infection.
5. Localized conjunctival hyperemia may point to an area of inflammation or damage on the cornea.

Once we know of any problems that will need to be managed, some background information is needed, if we do not already possess it.

The **current lens specification** is important, since if we do not know what the patient is using, we will not know how to improve on it. Reception staff should be trained to ask the patient to bring their specification with them to the appointment, as the Data Protection Act has made it difficult to gather information from previous practitioners on the day. We should also know the age of the current lenses, and the frequency of replacement suggested by the prescribing practitioner.

Previous contact lens history is of interest. If the patient has upgraded their lenses regularly as better ones have become available, it suggests that the general standard of care has been relatively high. Conversely, patients who are wearing lens designs of archaeological interest may be doing so through ignorance of anything better. Those patients who have changed their lens type may have done so in response to problems. The soft lens wearer who converts to silicone hydrogel lenses may have had significant neovascularization, and careful slit-lamp examination for ghost vessels is indicated. Where there is a history of repeated inflammatory or infective episodes, the likelihood is that the patient is more than usually prone to these events.

We should determine the **pattern of wear** in terms of the number of days per week and the hours per day that the lenses are worn, and whether this is imposed by choice or limited by problems.

The **care system** needs careful investigation, and several questions should be asked:

1. Which solutions are used? It is surprising how few patients actually know the correct name of the solution they are using, and it is useful to keep a few samples in the consulting room as an *aide-mémoire* ('it's that one in the blue bottle on the right').
2. Are these the ones that were prescribed by the practitioner? Surveys have shown that about one-third of patients are not using the solutions prescribed, and that the situation deteriorates with time. Patients change for a variety of reasons, including cost, availability, and simple curiosity. Some adopt a 'pick-and mix' approach, using a cleaner from one

manufacturer and a conditioning solution from another, and these solutions may not be compatible. Furthermore, if the preservatives are different, it can be time-consuming to identify the culprit in the event of solution sensitivity.

3. How old is the case? Patients have a habit of using a case well past its time, and this can interfere with the action of the solutions, and act as a significant source of infection, particularly as few patients clean them once the novelty of contact lens wear has worn off.

4. How do you use the solutions? It is best to watch the patient remove their lenses and then clean and disinfect as they normally would (assuming they would). This will give a valuable insight into their general approach to hygiene (did they wash their hands?), lens handling and use of solutions. Patients are often rather creative with solutions. Many clean the lenses before insertion rather than before overnight soaking. 'Topping-up' of storage solutions rather than replacement is often adopted as an economy measure, sometimes with unfortunate consequences.

5. Do you use a protein remover? Many patients who have been given protein removers forget to replace them once they run out, or only use them when the lenses start to feel a bit sticky. Infrequent use is ineffective, as denatured protein will not be removed effectively.

6. Have you had any problems with solutions in the past? This will tell us what to avoid in future, in case we need to change the solutions in the future.

Vision and over-refraction

In most cases, recording of the vision with each eye and binocularly can be followed by a simple spherical over-refraction. If the vision not correctable to the required standard, sphero-cylindrical refraction may be required. A pinhole can be a quick way to determine whether there is any residual refractive error, and the retinoscope may detect uncorrected astigmatism. It should not be forgotten that contact lens patients are not immune to binocular vision anomalies, and a patient who appears to have good visual acuity but who is unhappy with their vision may require binocular investigation.

Assessment of the lenses

The lenses should be examined in situ, first with white light and subsequently with cobalt blue light with fluorescein instilled.

White light investigation with diffuse light, and then focal light with an angled beam about 2 mm wide, is used to determine the state of the lens. Edge damage and surface deterioration should be apparent. The patient should then be invited to look down, and the upper lid should be raised by the practitioner. As the tear film dries, surface deposits will become apparent.

1. Protein tends to take on a dull, grayish appearance when dried.
2. Lipid deposits are shinier, and look 'greasy'.

Right-handed patients will sometimes present with the '**left-lens syndrome**'. The right lens is often cleaned first, and the second lens may not be cleaned quite so thoroughly. In time, a significantly higher level of deposition will be seen on the lens that is cleaned second.

The fit of the lenses is assessed as described in Chapter 3. Practitioners should resist the urge to fiddle with a fit that is not causing any clinical problems, in pursuit of a perfect fit. If we are going to change anything, there should always be some tangible benefit to the patient, who is probably going to be paying for the change.

The patient should then be asked to remove and store their lenses as normal, and their technique and the state of the case can be observed. Slit-lamp investigation of the patient's eyes can then proceed. This follows the same pattern as that described in Chapter 1, observing the adnexa, tear layer and cornea in sequence.

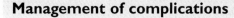

Management of complications

This is discussed in Chapter 9.

Promoting compliance

Many contact lens patients do not comply with their wearing schedules or care regimes. This is not a problem specific to contact lenses. Whenever human beings have devised substances or strategies of potential benefit to their fellows, other human beings have found ways of rendering them ineffective, or even dangerous. Non-compliance is not a product of the consumer age either. Hippocrates was moved to opine 'Patients are often lying when they say they have regularly taken their medicine.' This may seem a bit harsh, until we consider the facts. For short-term medication, such as a course of antibiotics, non-compliance rates of 20–30% are typical, rising to over 50% when the course of treatment is prolonged. The degree of obstinacy that patients may achieve is staggering. In one study, glaucoma patients were told that they would go blind if they did not comply with medication. Nevertheless, half of them did not comply often enough for treatment to be effective, and compliance did not improve even after sight was lost in one eye.

A study by Claydon and Efron (1994) gives us some interesting statistics. Twenty-seven percent of patients admitted to wearing their lenses for longer than instructed, and research conducted during the development of silicone hydrogel lenses suggests that many wear unsuitable lenses overnight at least occasionally, and this includes rigid gas permeable (RGP) lens wearers. It is also recognized that patients will seek to extend the lifespan of their lenses by using daily disposables for a week or more, and monthlies until they fall apart, often with inadequate care systems.

Claydon and Efron also found significant non-compliance with care systems. Sixty-two percent keep their solutions for too long, and many of these are probably 'topping-up' rather than replacing their solutions daily. Thirty-six percent clean their lenses only intermittently, and 8% not at all. Ten percent never rinse them. The relationship with tap water is fascinating. Three percent consider it a suitable medium for lens cleaning, yet 30% have such an aversion to it that they avoid washing their hands before handling their lenses.

The reasons for non-compliance are manifold. In some cases, the users may have been misinformed, either by a practitioner or by acquaintances, or they may have misunderstood the instructions. Simple ignorance should not be discounted. A Bausch & Lomb study found that 35% of patients thought that saline was for disinfection, and there is a story (possibly apocryphal) of a man who presented in the contact lens clinic of a leading hospital with the complaint that not only were his protein tablets ineffective but that he was sick every time he swallowed one. Cost cutting may motivate some non-compliant behavior. The patient who extends the lifespan of the lenses or of the solution may be trying to save money, but may equally be just too lazy to get some fresh products, and socio-economic status is a poor predictor of non-compliance.

The effect of boredom should not be ignored. Long-term therapy generally has higher non-compliance rates, and the situation deteriorates with the length of treatment. Contact lens care systems fall into the long-term category. Patients run out of a product, and either continue without it or use something else, perceived to be similar, until they can get to the supplier of the proper stuff. If no adverse effects occur immediately, they have little motivation to return to the original system, especially if the new version is cheaper or easier (and what could be cheaper and easier than doing nothing?). Some patients are simply curious. If they see a new product on the shelves of the supermarket, they simply have to try it, in the same way that they might try out a new shampoo, and advertising encourages such behavior. Finally, there may be some element of risk compensation involved. We live in a protected world, and some patients, particularly males, may incline towards risky behavior, consciously or subconsciously. After all, we smoke, drink, take recreational drugs and drive above the speed limit, sometimes all at once, despite well-publicized consequences.

Non-compliance may be sight-threatening. Even when the consequences are more trivial, they can waste a considerable amount of chair-time, especially as patients rarely make a full confession of their crimes at first. It is therefore essential that practitioners take steps to minimize it, although the statistics do not make encouraging reading.

Patients need to be aware that they are susceptible to complications as a result of non-compliance, and that these are not rare. Furthermore, the complications are sometimes severe and could result in blindness. Although the practitioner would not wish to terrify a patient unnecessarily, when one is faced with an individual whose ambitions appear to encompass the joys of microbial keratitis, some shock tactics may be in order. There are many pictures of microbial keratitis available these days, and a suitably gory example, kept on a practice computer or printed out, can concentrate the mind splendidly. Pick one with lots of red bits and purulent discharge for maximum effect. A short discussion of corneal grafts should complete the operation. For less severe transgressions, the carrot/stick ratio can be modified, by emphasizing the potential benefits for visual performance and comfort of compliant behavior.

Compliance may be aided by ensuring that the care system is simple and quick to use, and easily obtained. Novelty may promote at least short-term compliance, so there is a case for discussing new developments in both lenses and solutions at every aftercare visit. Free samples of new products are readily available to practitioners, and we should make use of them.

The one thing that is generally accepted to promote compliance is repetition. By reminding patients of the correct care regime at aftercare visits, Radford et al (1993) found that compliance rates could be raised from 44% to 90%. In summary, the strategy for promoting compliance should begin at the initial consultation and continue throughout the time that the patient continues to wear contact lenses.

1. At the initial visit, the practitioner must set an example by washing hands thoroughly before touching either the patient or a lens and by discussing the importance of hygiene and compliance.

2. During the collection appointment, clear information on the wearing and care of the lenses needs to be given verbally, although it would be optimistic to expect the patient to listen to it all. Many patients are in a rather nervous and excited state when first collecting their lenses, and much of the information goes in one ear and out of the other, without ever making any impression on the cognitive centers. For this reason, it is important to back any verbal information with a written version, as the odd patient may even read it. It is also useful to get the patient to sign a form acknowledging that a full discussion of the care of the lenses took place, as the patient's memory may be somewhat incomplete, especially if things subsequently go wrong.

3. The real work begins at the first aftercare visit. The patient should be asked to demonstrate their technique for removal, cleaning and storage of the lenses, and any deficiencies should be addressed. Many patients forget to wash their hands before removing the lenses, and this issue should be tackled at an early stage.

4. At subsequent aftercare visits, the same procedure should be adopted. We need to know what the patient is using, how they use it and how often they use it. The patient should also be made aware of any developments in lens design or solutions that might be of benefit to them. Too many patients gradually become out of date and eventually turn up for an infrequent aftercare visit wearing lenses that transmit little oxygen and that have been worn for too long, and with a care system that is either somewhat minimal or ill-matched to their lenses or wearing pattern. Such behavior becomes ingrained, and it can be difficult to convince this patient that change is a good thing. The patient who keeps his polymethyl methacrylate (PMMA) lenses on the bathroom shelf and licks them before insertion may prove to be particularly challenging, although it may be worth pointing out that the bacterial load would be lighter if he urinated on them instead.

5. Patients should be encouraged to make regular aftercare visits, at intervals of 6 months to a year, as longer periods encourage

non-compliance. Reminders should be sent out, and if they are not acted upon, attempts should be made to contact the patient. It may take time, but it will hopefully avoid the day when the patient turns up with a problem that takes weeks or months to resolve. Planned replacement of the contact lenses will tend to encourage regular attendance, as will the occasional upgrade. Continuity of care should also help in establishing trust between patient and practitioner.

6. It is important that the practitioner keeps abreast of new developments, as advertising in the media and on the internet is far more effective now than it used to be. A practitioner who knows less than the patient will rapidly lose all credibility and their advice will be ignored, probably with some justification. Regular continuing education and training (CET) and continuing professional development (CPD) is the remedy, and in the contact lens field the pace of change makes them essential.

References

Claydon BE and Efron N (1994) Non-compliance in contact lens wear. *Ophthal Physiol Opt* **14**: 356–364.

Radford CF, Woodward EG and Stapleton F (1993) Contact lens hygiene compliance in a university population. *J Br Contact Lens Assoc* **16**: 105–111.

Further reading

Sokol J, Meir MG and Bloom S (1990) A study of patient compliance in a contact lens wearing population. *Contact Lens Assoc Ophthalmol J* **16**: 209–213.

9
Complications and management

Introduction   136
Hypoxia   137
Drying   142
    Clinical signs   143
    Management   146
Mechanical insult   146
Toxic and hypersensitivity reactions   148
    Clinical signs   148
    Management   149
Sterile inflammation of the cornea   150
Infection   153
    Symptoms   156
    Clinical signs   156
Further reading   159

Introduction

Most aftercare appointments are fairly routine affairs, and as lens materials, lens designs and the care systems used with them have improved, some of the complications that were common have all but disappeared. Nevertheless, from time to time intervention is necessary to resolve problems that have arisen, and we can save time and money for both patient and practitioner by adopting a systematic approach. The strategy for effective management of complications involves the following steps:

1. Know your enemy. Correct identification of the root of the problem will save time and inconvenience. There is a tendency among those new to contact lens aftercare to bark up the wrong tree, often because of overreaction to a single clinical finding. Symptoms and signs are rarely solitary, and a single finding is rarely specific. The trick is to seek corroborative evidence. The more signs and symptoms that point to the same cause, the more likely it is that the diagnosis is accurate. There are 'families' of signs and symptoms, and the discovery of any family member should always prompt a thorough search for the parents and siblings. For soft contact lenses, the families are determined by the nature of the lenses themselves. They are plastic objects that sit on the eye, exerting pressure on the tear layer and cornea and restricting the availability of oxygen. They are accompanied by solutions and deposits that may cause toxic or hypersensitivity reactions. With that in mind, the families are as follows, although there is some overlap between them:
   (a) hypoxia
   (b) drying
   (c) mechanical insult
   (d) toxic and hypersensitivity reactions
   (e) sterile inflammation of the cornea
   (f) microbial keratitis.
2. Change one thing at a time, and see if it resolves the situation before making any more changes. A scattergun approach may

solve the problem at least as fast, but you will not know why. Should the problem recur, you will be none the wiser about what you need to do to tackle it.

3. Always keep in mind a worst case scenario for the signs and symptoms that you have collected, and an idea of the likely timescale involved. If this involves serious risk to the patient, as it will if microbial keratitis is suspected, make sure that you see the patient again before events can take their course. Bacterial ulcers become serious over hours rather than days, so seeing the patient in a week or so might be considered a little casual by a court of law.

4. Unless the worst case considerations are overriding, allow enough time for the changes to take effect. If the oxygen transmission is improved to eliminate microcysts, it makes little sense to see the patient in a fortnight, when the microcysts are certain to be more numerous. If the patient is seen in 3 months, you will be able to tell whether your management has worked.

5. Try not to 'bench-rest' patients. If a finding is not serious enough to do anything about, it will probably not be in a fortnight either. If the problem is too serious to ignore, it will probably not improve on its own, although there are always exceptions. Patients can usually tell when the practitioner is unsure, and a proactive approach with objectives that are clear to both parties is generally more reassuring. Recording these objectives on the clinical record is essential, and if instructions are lengthy, then it is worth considering writing them down for the patient.

Hypoxia

All contact lenses restrict the oxygen supply to some extent, although as lenses have developed over the years, the restriction has become much less, and the clinical signs rather more subtle, than in the old days of polymethyl methacrylate (PMMA), when every patient had central edema visible with the naked eye if the limbus was illuminated. The 'family' of signs and symptoms associated with hypoxia include the following.

Symptoms tend to be non-specific if mild, and patients will often complain of dryness when the actual cause is hypoxia. In more severe cases, the cornea may become edematous, leading to a loss of contrast and light scattering, which may cause photophobia towards the end of the wearing period. On the slit-lamp, the first sign may be **hyperemia** around the limbus. Corneal signs will depend on the severity of the condition. Visible areas of localized edema are rare in soft lens wearers, and more subtle signs should be sought. The signs are most likely to appear beneath the part of the lens that transmits the least oxygen, but they are often more easily detected in the central area against the dark background provided by the pupil. The degree of edema present at the time of examination may be indicated by the presence of striae and folds.

1. **Striae** are seen as fine, usually vertical, gray–white lines in the posterior stroma. They are best observed with direct illumination using a parallelepiped beam at about 16–20× magnification, against the background of the pupil area. Striae begin to appear when the level of edema reaches about 5%. In rigid gas permeable (RGP) lens wearers, they tend to appear in clusters rather than singly, if the level of edema is sufficiently high. They are probably caused by fluid separation of the collagen fibrils in the posterior stroma, which are predominantly vertically arranged.
2. **Folds** can be observed in the endothelial mosaic using specular reflection, appearing as grooves and ridges. If severe, they may appear as dark branching lines under direct illumination. They are caused by buckling of the posterior stroma with high levels of edema. They appear when the level of edema is about 15%, and the cornea is likely to be somewhat hazy when in this state.

Acute hypoxia is probably less significant than **chronic hypoxia**, and the latter may be detected by the following clinical signs:

1. **Epithelial microcysts** and **vacuoles** appear as small gray dots in the epithelium under direct illumination (Fig. 9.1).

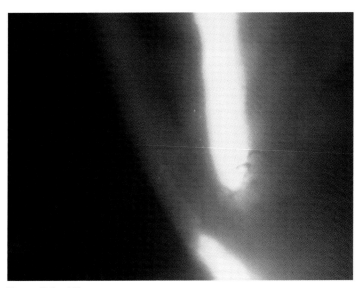

Figure 9.1 Microcysts

Initially, they may be difficult to distinguish from dust particles
in the tear film, but if the patient blinks, they are the ones
that do not move. The best way to identify them is to use
an angled parallelepiped beam at high (40×) magnification.
The area of cornea to observe is that where the indirectly
illuminated and retroilluminated areas meet, i.e. in **marginal
retroillumination**.

2. Microcysts, because they have a higher refractive index than
   the surrounding tissue, show reversed illumination under these
   conditions and may appear as tiny pinpricks. Vacuoles are
   generally slightly larger and do not show reversed illumination,
   so they appear as small bubbles. They represent fluid collected
   in the intracellular spaces, and are therefore indicative of
   edema, which may be caused by hypoxia or hypertonic ocular
   exposure. It is possible that these intercellular spaces are
   exploited by *Acanthamoeba* to gain access to the cornea, so the
   presence of significant numbers should not be tolerated. Some
   patients may have a few of these independent of contact lens

wear. Microcysts are probably apoptotic (i.e. dead) cells that are either ingested by phagocytes or encapsulated by material from the basement membrane and eventually expelled after traveling through the corneal layers. They are probably created by a combination of hypoxia, which produces lactic acid, and hypercapnia (increase in carbon dioxide levels), which produces carbonic acid. They may also be induced by mechanical trauma in some cases. They can be eliminated by improving the level of oxygen available, but the recovery process is unusual. Initially, the number of microcysts will increase, as the corneal metabolism speeds up and cellular debris is removed more efficiently. There is then a gradual decrease in the number until they are finally eliminated. This can take 3–5 months. The point at which microcysts become significant is subjective, but generally, if staining is also present, intervention is required.

3. Changes to the endothelium may also occur in response to the acidosis caused by hypoxia and hypercapnia. An acute response is observed in all contact lens wearers within a few minutes of lens insertion. When the endothelium is observed by specular reflection, a number of dark areas can be observed within the endothelial mosaic. These are **blebs**, and represent swollen cells that disrupt the smooth mirror-like surface of the endothelium–aqueous interface. After 20–30 minutes, the number of blebs peaks, and it then falls over the next hour, although some blebs will be visible throughout the wearing period. The chronic response to acidosis is polymegathism, where the cells of the endothelial mosaic appear to vary markedly in size. **Polymegathism** occurs naturally with age, so the endothelium should be judged against expectations for a given age group. It is not easy to assess the endothelium accurately with a slit-lamp. The highest magnification available is usually 40× or less, and even at 40× with a good slit-lamp the best that can be seen is a textured area, and only the more advanced degrees of polymegathism may be detected with any reliability. This is most likely to be seen with low-Dk lenses, especially 38% hydroxyethylmethacrylate (HEMA), and in hydrogel extended wear lenses. Polymegathism is a response to significant metabolic stress, and remedial action should be

taken if it is detected. Recovery is at best very slow, and may not occur at all.

4. **Neovascularization** is a common finding in soft lens wearers. Up to half a millimeter of vessel growth is commonly seen as a physiologic response to lens wear and need not necessarily lead to greater vessel growth. To those unused to contact lens aftercare, half a millimeter can look quite frightening under high magnification, and it is useful to measure the true extent of the vessels either by reference to a graticule in the eyepiece of the slit-lamp or by comparing the vessels with the overlap of the lens beyond the limbus. This is typically 1–1.5 mm, depending upon the horizontal visible iris diameter (HVID) of the patient and the total diameter of the lens. It is important to determine whether we are looking at a condition that is active, static or receding. The presence of limbal hyperemia is a useful clue, as an eye with undilated limbal arcades is less likely to be under hypoxic stress. Neovascularization is an inflammatory process, and the presence of diffuse infiltrates around the leading vessels is not a good sign. Conversely, the presence of 'ghost vessels' would suggest that the cornea is currently receiving adequate oxygen.

Significant chronic hypoxia is known to increase the risk of microbial keratitis, and it is now easy to address. The management of hypoxia consists, not surprisingly, of arranging for greater oxygen availability. This may be achieved in the following ways:

1. Wearing the lenses less. This may be effective in the short term, but rarely in the longer term. The wearing pattern that a patient adopts is largely dictated by convenience for that individual, and the patient will probably return to their previous wearing pattern sooner rather than later.
2. Improving the flow of tears under the lens may improve oxygen levels to a limited extent. A smaller total diameter, greater edge lift and smoother transitions may bring some improvement.
3. By far the most effective strategy is to use a more permeable material. There are materials available now that have sufficient

permeability to eliminate the sign of hypoxia in any normal cornea. It should be borne in mind that if microcysts are being used as an indicator, refitting with a high-Dk material will initially increase the number, so an aftercare interval of about 3 months is useful unless contraindicated by other clinical concerns.

Drying

Many patients complain of symptoms of dryness, but not all of them are actually due to drying. Considerable research has been undertaken with a view to improve the wetting performance of contact lenses in recent years, but the improvement in patient satisfaction, while considerable, has been less than perhaps anticipated. What patients are actually complaining of is persistent, progressive mild irritation and lens awareness, and this

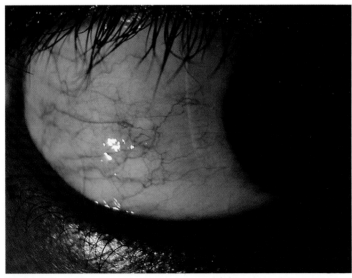

Figure 9.2   Bulbar hyperemia

could be due to hypoxia or mild inflammation rather than drying per se.

Drying can cause lens awareness or discomfort, and this usually worsens progressively throughout the wearing time. The vision is often variable, due to the accumulation of deposits on the lens, and again this gets worse towards the end of the wearing period. The other frequent patient complaint is of red eyes, and characteristically this is associated with hyperemia of the bulbar conjunctiva in the area exposed between the lid margins (Fig. 9.2).

Clinical signs

The clinical signs to look for include the following.

Anomalies of the lid margin are best viewed by diffuse illumination under fairly low magnification and they may give a clue to the underlying cause of the problem. **Blepharitis**, which can be associated with changes in both conjunctiva and cornea, may cause an unstable tear film that could affect contact lens wear. Chronic blepharitis may be encountered as the anterior form, either staphylococcal or sebborrheic. There is also a posterior type, also known as meibomian gland dysfunction (MGD).

The **staphylococcal** form tends to be seen in patients with atopic eczema and is more common in females and young patients. The lid margins are hyperemic and show telangiectases (dilated, tortuous blood vessels). There is also scaling. The scales are brittle, and form collarettes around the bases of the lashes. Where they have been removed, small bleeding ulcers may be seen. This condition is caused by chronic staphylococcal infection of the bases of the lashes, so any patient with it has an increased bacterial load. It should be eliminated before contact lens wear is allowed. Complications that may be observed include whitening or complete loss of the lashes and trichiasis. The lid margins may become scarred and notched. If the infection spreads to the glands of Zeis and Moll, a stye may be the result. If the meibomian glands become involved, there may be an internal hordeolum. Acute bacterial conjunctivitis may appear, and recur. Apart from these direct bacterial effects, the exotoxins released by the bacteria may cause hypersensitivity reactions. A mild papillary conjunctivitis, marginal corneal infiltrates or, rarely, phlyctenulosis and pannus may occur. About half of all sufferers also have an unstable tear film. Management consists of lid scrubs and referral to a general practitioner for antibiotics and possibly anti-inflammatory agents.

The **seborrheic** version tends to associated with seborrheic dermatitis, which can affect the scalp, face and chest. There is an oily type in which the scaling is greasy, and also a dry type (dandruff). The symptoms are similar to, although milder than, those of the staphylococcal form. The hyperemia and telangiectasia of the lid margins are also more moderate, and the scales are greasy and yellowish, and do not leave an ulcer when removed. The lids may be greasy and stuck together. There may be a moderate papillary conjunctivitis and punctate keratitis, which tends to favor the middle third of the cornea, whereas the staphylococcal form often affects the lower third of the cornea. Management usually involves lid scrubs, using sodium bicarbonate or baby shampoo as a degreasing agent.

Posterior blepharitis (MGD) may be divided into meibomian seborrhea and meibomitis. Meibomian seborrhea causes hypersecretion from dilated meibomian glands. The lid margins may show small oil globules or waxy collections. The tear film may be oily and foamy, and in severe cases there may be a frothy discharge at the inner canthus (meibomian foam). The patient complains of burning eyes on first waking, and there may be few signs of inflammation, so this is easy to miss. If the lid margins are gently squeezed, copious discharge may be elicited. It should be remembered that the lid margins are sensitive, and the expression of meibomian contents usually hurts, especially when attempted by the inexperienced. It is therefore not a procedure to be recommended for an asymptomatic patient.

Primary meibomitis involves inflammation centered around the orifices of the meibomian glands, which may pout and be capped by domes of oily material (meibomana). Expressed meibomian contents are thickened and may contain more solid particles, in some cases resembling toothpaste, and requiring firm pressure to express. If the contents become trapped, meibomian cysts may form. Papillary conjunctivitis and punctate epitheliopathy may be secondary effects. About one-third of these patients have tear film instability. Meiobomitis may also occur with secondary seborrheic blepharitis, associated with seborrheic dermatitis, the meibomian involvement usually being relatively mild and patchy. Management involves lid scrubs and referral to the general practitioner for oral antibiotics, typically tetracycline. Treatment may take 3 months or more.

The contact lenses are likely to have heavy deposits of protein, lipid or both. The exact nature of the deposits will depend on individual tear chemistry, the lens material and the solution being used. If the upper lid is held by the practitioner, and the patient instructed to look down, the surface of the lens will dry. Protein deposits tend to have a dull, grayish appearance, whereas lipid deposits are shinier. The pre-lens tear film is likely to be unstable.

Following lens removal, other signs may be apparent:

1. The tear break-up time (TBUT) may be low, often below 10 seconds, and the tear layer will appear foamy or 'bitty'.

2. The bulbar conjunctiva will be hyperemic, sometimes in a band from inner to outer canthus. Frequently, there will be marked conjunctival fluorescein staining in the same area. In severe cases, a wing-shaped vascular lesion may encroach upon the cornea from the conjunctiva. This is **pseudopterygium** rather than true pterygium, which is a degenerative condition, although it may look similar.

3. There may be corneal staining. Typically this involves the lower part of the cornea, often in an arcuate pattern referred to as 'smile stain'. Smile stain is caused by evaporation of fluid through the lens secondary to localized desiccation on the surface. Eventually, the corresponding area of post-lens tear film becomes exhausted, and mechanical abrasion of the corneal surface occurs. Usually, this appears as mild punctate stain, and in this form it is a common finding in thin, disposable lenses, particularly in the summer months. In severe cases, the staining may become confluent, and this will carry an increased risk of infection. In such cases, suspension of lens wear to clear the staining should precede refitting with a lens less likely to dry out.

Management

Management of dryness can involve a number of strategies:

1. Elimination of causative factors, especially the various forms of blepharitis, should be pursued. Lid scrubs and hot compresses will be useful for MGD and seborrheic anterior blepharitis, while staphylococcal blepharitis will need antimicrobial treatment, which may require routine referral to a general practitioner. However, if the dryness of the eyes is caused by systemic medication or a medical condition, elimination of the cause may be outside the control of the contact lens practitioner.

2. Careful selection of care systems may help to reduce or remove deposits. Lipid deposits are often seen with solutions containing chlorhexidene. Protein deposition may require the use of an enzyme cleaner. Compliance with cleaning regimes should also be encouraged.

3. Old lenses tend to deposit more, so planned replacement may help considerably, particularly as modern materials tend to scratch more easily.

4. The use of certain materials may improve comfort considerably as well as reducing deposition.

5. If all else fails, rewetting or 'comfort' drops may relieve symptoms. However, they are rarely a long-term solution, as patients eventually either stop using them or use them so infrequently that they make little difference. In the past, a few patients went to the other extreme, instilling preserved comfort drops in large amounts and eventually becoming allergic to them.

Mechanical insult

A number of symptoms caused by mechanical insult may be seen:

1. Steep lenses may trap small bubbles under the optic zone. These can cause small circular depressions in the cornea, which may retain fluorescein, although the epithelial surface is

intact. With the major slit-lamp it looks like rather coarse, and neatly circular, punctate staining. This **dimple veiling** is usually asymptomatic, although if it is severe some visual degradation may be noticed. A flatter fit, increased edge lift or smoother transitions will generally eliminate it. Dimple veiling can also be associated with **mucin balls**. These are created by sheer forces acting on the mucin component of the tears, and with the lens in place they appear as small gray bodies between the back surface of the lens and the cornea. They rarely cause problems but there are reports of a correlation between mucin balls and an increased frequency of inflammatory events.

2. **Superior epithelial arcuate lesions** (SEALs) may appear in the upper, and occasionally lower, cornea as arcuate areas of confluent staining. They appear to be more common in patients wearing the 'stiffer' silicone hydrogel lenses than in those wearing hydrogel lenses, leading to the conclusion that most SEALs are caused by mechanical forces under the lens. However, many other factors have been associated with SEALs over the years, including tight lids, hypoxia and solution reactions. The patient may be asymptomatic or have mild discomfort. If lens wear is suspended for 2 weeks, symptoms will resolve in about half of the patients and are unlikely to recur on resumption of wear. However, the rest of the patients will need refitting, often with a 'softer' lens. Unfortunately, only about half of these patients will have resolution of symptoms, and suspension of lens wear may be necessary, given that SEALs represent a significant epithelial defect.

3. Mechanical irritation may also induce **papillary conjunctivitis** in silicone hydrogel lens wearers, usually of the upper lid. The earliest sign is hyperemia of the upper palpebral conjunctiva relative to the conjunctiva of the lower lid, although this may be asymptomatic. Later, papillae will appear, and may coalesce to form giant papillae with diameters over 1 mm. The papillae themselves are hyperplastic vascular tissue and have a central vascular core. Should the papillae become inflamed, the lens may adhere to them and decenter, creeping up under the lid. It may also be caused by an immune response to deposits on the lens, and this is thought to be the more

common etiology in hydrogel lens wearers. Management will depend on the perceived cause. Mechanical papillary conjunctivitis may be tackled by improving the edge profile, reducing edge stand-off by changing the total diameter or reducing edge lift in one or more meridians. That due to deposits may be improved by more effective cleaning and frequent lens replacement. The use of non-preserved care systems may also useful in these cases.

4. Patients may present at aftercare appointments with staining in the 4 and 8 o'clock positions that can sometimes extend across the whole lower cornea, thus mimicking drying stain. This may indicate mechanical abrasion caused by a clumsy lens removal technique, whereby the lens is pinched straight off the cornea rather than moving down on to the sclera first.

Toxic and hypersensitivity reactions

Intolerance to solutions is considerably less common than was once the case, due to improvements in their formulation, particularly the preservative elements. However, they are still encountered from time to time. Some become apparent within a day or two of first use of the solution, but there are occasions when the symptoms gradually build up over a period of time before they become severe enough for the patient to consult their practitioner. Early clinical signs may be apparent in an asymptomatic patient. The symptoms associated with solution intolerance are typically noticed immediately after the lenses are inserted, and may resolve if the lenses are kept in and the solutions diluted by the tear film. Lens awareness, itching, burning and sensations of dryness are all common. In severe cases, photophobia may be reported.

Clinical signs

The clinical signs may include the following in patients with mild or no symptoms:

1. Hyperemia of the palpebral and bulbar conjunctiva. The latter may have a diffuse pattern that is more marked around the limbus.
2. Superficial punctate keratitis. This may favor the lower cornea, but is typically diffused over the corneal surface.
3. Occasionally, infiltrates may be observed. These are usually intraepithelial or subepithelial. They may be discrete or diffuse, and tend to favor the area just inside the limbus.

More severe reactions will have symptoms, sometimes quite marked, and the following signs may be present:

1. The lids may be swollen.
2. The tear film may be unstable, and mucus strands may be visible. Reflex lacrimation is common.
3. Conjunctival hyperemia.
4. Diffuse superficial punctate keratitis.
5. In hypersensitivity reactions, infiltrates may be observed, although there is usually a delay of about 24 hours between the initial signs and symptoms and the appearance of infiltrates.

Management

The management of solution reactions will depend on their severity. If the symptoms and signs are severe, it is wise to suspend contact lens wear until the eye returns to normal, especially as the signs of microbial infection may be rather similar. If there is any question of infection, the patient should be seen the next day. Once the initial reaction has subsided, or if the clinical signs are mild to begin with, management involves identifying likely triggering agents and avoiding them. The prime suspect in these cases is usually the preservative in the conditioning solution. However, a surprising number of patients clean their lenses before insertion, and may not rinse them thoroughly before insertion, so the cleaning solution may also be a factor to consider. Buffering agents and residues from enzymatic systems may also be suspected on occasion. Careful questioning of the patient is necessary to establish precisely what solutions are in use, and how they are used. It may not even be the solutions used for the lenses, as self-prescribed or general practitioner-prescribed eye-drops can cause the same reactions. Where more than one potential suspect is present, eliminate them one at a time, in descending order of probability, until the signs and symptoms are eliminated. Strictly speaking, a causal relationship can only be proven by reintroducing the suspected agent and observing the return of clinical signs. However, this may be a test too far for most contact lens wearers, so this step is usually omitted.

Sterile inflammation of the cornea

Inflammation of the cornea is not specific to one causative agent. The same response will occur whatever the initial trigger. The trigger can be trauma, toxicity or immune response, and the common factor is that corneal cells, usually in the epithelium, become distressed and release chemical agents that initiate the inflammatory response. Contact lens wear tends to potentiate all of the likely triggers:

1. **Trauma** is more likely as the cornea may be hypoxic, which makes the epithelium more fragile and slow to repair. Insertion and removal of the lenses may induce mechanical insult.
2. Contact lens solutions, deposits and bacterial toxins are all capable of inducing a **toxic response**. In extended wear, the products of dead epithelial cells may also be a source, as they may be trapped under the lens for some time. Immobile lenses may keep the dead cells in one location, which will increase the likelihood of localized epithelial distress.
3. Solution deposits and bacterial toxins may also cause immune responses, and the cornea may also react to chemicals released by adjacent inflamed tissues, such as the palpebral conjunctiva. Infiltrates are sometimes noted as an 'innocent bystander' effect of contact lens-related papillary conjunctivitis (CLPC).

Inflammation consists of four classic elements, Rubor, Calor, Tumor and Dolor. Vascular dilation causes:

1. rubor (redness or hyperemia)
2. calor (increase in temperature.

Increased vascular permeability results in:

1. tumor (swelling, edema)
2. dolor (discomfort and pain).

In the anterior eye, these signs are often fairly subtle unless the response is severe, and a severe response always suggests the possibility of infection. In the cornea, the most useful sign of inflammation is the presence of infiltrates, which are collections of white blood cells. These may form discrete patches or diffuse areas in the epithelium and anterior stroma. Generally speaking, the more serious the cause, the deeper they are and the more likely they are to be central, but this is only a rough guide.

Clinically, corneal infiltrates can be divided into the following categories, in ascending order of seriousness:

1. asymptomatic infiltrates
2. asymptomatic infiltrative keratitis
3. infiltrative keratitis
4. contact lens-associated red eye (CLARE)
5. contact lens peripheral ulcer (CLPU)
6. microbial keratitis (see Infection, p.153).

Asymptomatic infiltrates are sometimes seen in non-contact lens wearers (about 5%), and are probably unrelated to contact lens wear, as they have a similar incidence in contact lens wearers. They may be induced by environmental factors such as air pollution. Typically, there are one or more small (up to 0.2 mm), discrete, grayish-white patches anywhere on the cornea. These are intraepithelial or occasionally subepithelial (an optical section at high magnification will indicate how deep the infiltrate is). There are no symptoms or other signs of inflammation. No action is required.

In **asymptomatic infiltrative keratitis** there is a diffuse infiltrate in the peripheral parts of the cornea, sometimes with some discrete infiltrates as well. It does not appear to cause any problems in itself, but it may be a mild form of CLARE, with similar causes, so the patient's care of the lenses should be under scrutiny.

Infiltrative keratitis can present as a diffuse or focal infiltrate, but here it is accompanied by symptoms of discomfort or pain, and by bulbar conjunctival hyperemia, especially around the limbal area. The focal form is probably a response to local epithelial trauma caused by a foreign body trapped under an immobile lens. The diffuse form may be a mild form of CLARE response, with similar etiology.

CLARE itself is a complication of extended wear, and typically the onset is in the early hours of the morning, after a period when the eyes have been closed. It is less common with RGP lenses than with soft lenses, but it has been reported with bound, immobile lenses. There is an association with Gram-negative bacteria, as about one-third of people with CLARE have contaminated lenses. The symptoms vary from mild discomfort to pain, and there is marked bulbar hyperemia, especially around the limbus. Feint diffuse infiltrates are seen arising from the limbal arcades, although there may be focal infiltrates present as well. Following a CLARE reaction, fine keratic precipitates (bedewing) may appear on the corneal endothelium. These are the result of mild anterior chamber activity and persist for about 6 months, so they can be a useful clue to past inflammatory events that the patient may not report.

CLPU presents as a round or oval grayish-white infiltrate with an overlying full-thickness epithelial defect. It is generally located near the periphery of the cornea, although there is a band of clear cornea between the infiltrate and the limbus. It may be asymptomatic or painful. Hyperemia may be generalized or limited to an area adjacent to the lesion. It is culture negative, although a correlation has been found with high levels of Gram-positive bacteria. If lens wear is suspended, signs and symptoms will resolve in 48 hours, except for the infiltrate, which can persist for up to 3 months, although it usually resolves within 1 month. It is likely that the infiltrate represents a response to localized trauma or toxicity and that the epithelial loss is a result of leukocyte action. However, given the epithelial defect and the bacterial correlation, caution is advisable, and the patient should be seen the next morning if they are not referred.

The management of sterile inflammation depends on its severity, and upon the chances that it might be an infection. The asymptomatic and white-eyed forms generally need no intervention, although CLARE's smaller sisters might be regarded as a warning shot from the bacteria, and lens hygiene might be worth some scrutiny. The symptomatic forms will require suspension of lens wear. This should ideally be until infiltrates have resolved, unless we are sure that the cause is unthreatening. The time required will vary with the location and depth of the infiltrate. Intraepithelial infiltrates resolve within 2–3 weeks, but subepithelial and anterior stromal infiltrates take longer, up to 3 months in some cases. Anything that persists longer than that in the absence of active inflammation is probably a scar, and these tend to have a 'bull's-eye' appearance, with a fainter center.

Infection

The eye may be infected by viruses, fungi, bacteria and amebae, but it is only the latter two that can be considered contact lens complications. Wearers may present with viral or fungal infection, but it is unlikely that the contact lenses played a significant part in the etiology. However, in bacterial and ameboidal infection, contact lens wear is a significant risk factor, and the majority of patients presenting at eye casualty departments for these conditions are contact lens wearers. The precise incidence of microbial keratitis is difficult to pin down, since cultures are unreliable and many patients are treated as infectious cases on appearance rather than waiting for the unpleasant later stages to confirm the diagnosis. An incidence of around 0.5% has been suggested for soft lenses worn on a daily basis, although extended wear figures are about six times higher.

Contact lenses modify the flushing action of the tears, and may change the mucin layer of the tear film. They restrict the oxygen supply to a greater or lesser extent. A hypoxic epithelium is less resistant to abrasion and takes longer to repair. Microorganisms adhere more easily to the cornea when oxygen levels are low. Finally, both the contact lenses and the storage case may be carrying far more microorganisms than would normally be present in the eye. The most common infections by far are bacterial. In non-contact lens wearers, Gram-positive bacteria such as *Staphylococcus* are the most common ocular infectious agents, but contact lens wear appears to favor Gram-negative bacteria, particularly *Pseudomonas aeruginosa*. The fact that the active form of *Acanthamoeba* feeds on Gram-negative bacteria may suggest why it is almost exclusively a problem encountered in contact lens wearers.

The **PEDAL** (Pain, Epithelial defect, Discharge, Anterior chamber activity, Location) mnemonic is widely used when attempting to differentiate between sterile and microbial (especially bacterial) keratitis. However, in contact lens wearers it has some limitations:

1. **Pain** may vary considerably between individuals, but in general, the worse it is, the more likely it is that we are dealing with an infection. However, there are some patients whose corneal sensitivity is reduced (patients with corneal fatigue and those who have had corneal surgery).

2. An **epithelial defect** overlying an infiltrate is always worrying, although it may be caused by the actions of white blood cells rather than by an infecting microbe. However, many 'sterile' inflammations are associated with bacterial toxins, and the combination of high levels of bacteria and a breached epithelium is one that leaves considerable scope for secondary infection.

3. **Discharge** is rather variable. *Staphylococcus* may produce little or no discernable discharge. *Streptococcus* and the Gram-negative bacteria tend to be fairly gooey, and gonorrhea highly productive.

4. **Anterior chamber activity** should always be present during active ulceration but it varies from a trace to dense flare and cells. Sterile lesions (e.g. CLARE) may also be associated with a moderate anterior chamber reaction.

5. **Location** is also somewhat unreliable in contact lens wearers. In non-wearers, ulcers tend to favor the central areas of the cornea, remote from the limbal vasculature. However, this is not the case in contact lens wearers, as their corneas are more likely to have physical damage peripherally, and the virulent organisms involved are able to overcome ocular defenses. For a contact lens wearer, any suspicious staining lesion in the central area is quite possibly an ulcer, but more peripheral ones could be.

When attempting to diagnose a **bacterial infection**, it is useful to consider **risk factors**. Contact lens-related factors include:

1. non-compliance with care regimes
2. poor hygiene
3. lens binding
4. extended wear
5. old lenses (>6 months)
6. dirty lenses
7. dirty case.

In addition, there are some **health-related factors** that will increase the chances of infection:

1. diabetes
2. travel to a warm climate
3. staphylococcal toxins (blepharitis and marginal infiltrates)
4. dry eyes
5. immunocompromised patients (e.g. AIDS patients or those on immunosuppressants)
6. postsurgical corneas
7. use of topical steroids
8. corneal trauma.

In general, it is thought that bacteria are unable to infect a cornea with an intact epithelium, although some strains of *Pseudomonas* are capable of this in laboratory conditions at least.

The signs and symptoms of bacterial infection are a combination of effects attributable to the organism and its associated toxins and those produced by the opposing defense mechanisms, which may in some cases be rather worse.

Symptoms

Symptoms may vary according to individual tolerance, but include (in approximate ascending order of seriousness):

1. irritation or lens awareness
2. burning sensation often associated with bacterial toxins
3. lacrimation
4. photophobia secondary to edema
5. reduced visible aperture secondary to edema and infiltration
6. foreign body sensation, especially if it increases upon lens removal
7. dull, aching pain due to inflammation and uveal involvement.

Clinical signs

Clinical signs will also vary according to the bacterial strain involved. They include the following:

1. The lids may be swollen and a pseudoptosis maybe present.
2. The palpebral conjunctiva will have a red, 'meaty' appearance and papillae.
3. Mucopurulent discharge will be present in the tears, especially with streptococcal and Gram-negative bacterial infection.
4. The bulbar conjunctiva will be purplish-red and often swollen. Hemorrhages are sometimes seen with streptococcal and Gram-negative infections.

5. Corneal ulceration destroys the epithelium and underlying stroma, producing a depressed lesion. This may be clearly defined (typical of streptococci) or indistinct around the edges, and the margins may show an overhang of tissue. Fluorescein stain will pool in the depression and fluoresce brightly but will then spread into the stroma amorphously within minutes.

6. A lesion over 2 mm in diameter should be regarded as microbial, but they all have to start somewhere, and smaller lesions should not be discounted on dimensions alone.

7. The corneal stroma will become edematous, often involving more than 50% of the area and depth.

8. Infiltration will be deep, sometimes full thickness, and will be seen as a hazy or opaque area. Occasionally, a deep ring infiltrate is seen with *Pseudomonas*.

9. Stromal abscess, stromal melting and perforation can occur with virulent forms, sometimes within a day or two.

10. Anterior chamber activity may range from very mild to severe cells and flare, sometimes forming a hypopyon in the anterior chamber. The intraocular pressure may increase secondary to anterior chamber involvement, although it might be a bit of a challenge to measure it.

11. The pupil is often miotic.

12. Neovascularization may occur if treatment is delayed.

13. Scarring of the corneal stroma is more or less inevitable.

The time it takes for things to get serious will vary with the organism involved, but the more virulent forms of *Pseudomonas* can cause severe scarring or perforation in a day or two. With this in mind, if corneal infection is suspected, it is wise to see the patient the next day, preferably in the morning, if you have not already referred them to eye casualty. If there is more than a suspicion, this should be treated as an ocular emergency and referred without delay.

Acanthamoeba is a common protozoan that occasionally produces severe corneal problems, almost invariably in contact lens wearers. It exists in both an active trophozoite form and as an inert, highly resistant cyst. Although most often associated with soft lenses, *Acanthamoeba* keratitis has been found in RGP lens wearers. It is known that exposure to stagnant water sources will increase risk, and these include swimming pools, hot tubs and the domestic hot water supply. (The relatively high incidence in the UK may be related to the common use of standing domestic water supplies in water tanks in the loft.) There is often, but not always, a history of corneal trauma.

The symptoms are not specific to *Acanthamoeba*, but the pain reported is often far more dramatic than the clinical findings would suggest.

Early clinical signs include the following:

1. Swollen lids.
2. Perilimbal hyperemia.
3. Staining at this stage is often minimal, but it fails to respond to standard anti-infective regimes.

Later signs include the following:

1. Corneal infiltrates, which tend to mimic those of other conditions, leading to misdiagnosis. They may be nummular, mimicking adenovirus, or pseudodendritic in form, which may lead to a diagnosis of herpes simplex or herpes zoster infection. Other 'viral' signs such as pseudomembranes and pre-auricular adenopathy may be present. Any patient diagnosed with these conditions who fails to respond to treatment may have *Acanthamoeba* keratitis.
2. Perilimbal infiltrates are specific to *Acanthamoeba*, and may account for the excessive pain associated with this condition.
3. A ring infiltrate or ulcer will eventually form. Stromal melt and perforation are possible.
4. Anterior chamber activity may be marked, and hypopyon and scleral melt are possible.

The condition advances slowly in comparison to bacterial events, often with remissions. It is difficult to identify positively, and treatment is often initiated ex juvantia (i.e. when other therapy has failed). When correct treatment is initiated, it may take months to resolve and the prognosis may be poor.

Where *Acanthamoeba* is suspected (and it should always be suspected if the pain is disproportionate to the clinical signs, or if the condition has failed to resolve as expected), prompt referral is indicated. As a temporary measure, brolene has been found to have a limited action against the active form.

Further reading

Brennan NA and Bruce AS (1997) *A Guide to Clinical Contact Lens Management.* CIBA Vision Corp.: Oxford.

Catania LJ (1998) *Primary Care of the Anterior Segment*, 2nd edn. Appleton and Lange: Norwalk, CT.

Jones LW and Jones DA (2000) *Common Contact Lens Complications.* Butterworth-Heinmann: Oxford.

Silbert JA (2000) *Anterior Segment Complications of Contact Lens Wear.* Butterworth-Heinmann: Boston, MA.

Tomlinson A (1992) *Complications of Contact Lens Wear.* Mosby Year Book: St Louis.

10
Tinted and therapeutic lenses

Introduction   162
Cosmetic lenses   162
UV-absorbing lenses   165
Therapeutic lenses   166
Further reading   169

Introduction

Soft contact lenses may be tinted for a number of reasons:

1. 'Handling tints' make the lens more visible against a white background, so they are easier to find in the case, or if they are dropped onto a work surface or sink. This works rather less well if the background surface is itself colored, of course.
2. Cosmetic lenses are used to modify or change the appearance of the eyes.
3. UV-blocking lenses reduce the levels of UVA and UVB radiation reaching the retina and lens.
4. Sports tints have recently been introduced to assist performance in sports such as golf and shooting.

Cosmetic lenses

Colored contact lenses allow a patient to modify or completely change the appearance of their eyes. In the USA, about 8% of soft lens wearers have colored lenses, although in Europe the figure is lower, around 6%; however, one in five adults in the UK say that they would consider trying them. The majority of these are young, between 16 and 35 years of age, which suggests that a significant part of the motivation is concerned with finding a mate. Many of those who do not require visual correction wear plano colored lenses purely for cosmetic reasons. Until recently, the supply of plano lenses was effectively unrestricted, as they were not classified as optical appliances under UK or US law. Hairdressers, beauty salons and clothes shops all supplied these lenses, and mail-order and internet sources were also active. There were reports of wearers sharing and exchanging lenses, and many of the outlets failed to give adequate advice on lens care and hygiene. Not surprisingly, reports of microbial keratitis soon followed. In the UK, plano cosmetic lenses are now effectively under the same legislation as other lenses, in that they can only be supplied to a specification issued by a registered medical practitioner, optometrist or dispensing optician, and the seller must make arrangements to provide reasonable aftercare. Similar legislation will be implemented in the USA.

The psychology of eye color is complex. In a survey of American women, respondents were given a set of eight attributes – creative, devious, kind, intelligent, sexy, shy, sweet and trustworthy – that they were asked to attribute to various eye colors. Blue eyes were most associated with sweet (42%), sexy (21%) and kind (10%). Green eyes were associated with sexy (29%), creative (25%) and devious (20%). Brown eyes were associated with intelligent (34%), trustworthy (16%) and kind (13%). It should be stressed that there is considerable variation between individuals and that the survey was of an ethnically and culturally diverse sample, with 29% blue eyes, 29% green and 42% brown, with the rest having eyes described as honey, gray, turquoise and amethyst. It would seem, then, that a certain eye color could emphasize certain desirable traits in an individual on first acquaintance. There is also the desire to stand out in a crowd. In countries where darker irides are usually associated with darker skin tones, green or blue eyes may be striking, and the use of 'fun' lenses with patterns with deliberately unnatural colors or patterns may well break the ice at parties. Carefully chosen, colored lenses may have the desired effect, but there is also a potential for 'fashion disasters' that leave the wearer looking ill, or a little demented.

Cosmetic lenses may be divided into three main categories:

1. 'Enhancers' are translucent lenses that allow the natural iris color to show through. Light incident on the iris is scattered by the iris stroma. Short-wavelength light is absorbed by the chromatophores within the stroma. Blue eyes have relatively few chromatophores, so more light is reflected back towards an observer. An enhancer lens placed on a blue eye will modify the spectrum of light incident on the iris, and because quite a lot of it is reflected back, a marked effect on iris color will be observed. With darker eyes, little of the incident light is reflected, so the effect of an enhancer tint will be marginal.

2. Opaque tints act as the main reflecting surface, so they have more effect on the iris appearance, whatever the underlying color. Solid opaque tints give a strange, doll-like appearance to the eyes, so most have an iris pattern incorporated, sometimes in more than one color.

3. 'Fun' or 'crazy' lenses are not designed to be natural. They are opaque lenses with patterns or pictures that make a statement, sometimes showing allegiance to a sports team or socio-political message.

Translucent tints may be created by four basic methods:

1. Dye dispersion, where the tint is added to the lens polymer, is mostly used on rigid gas permeable (RGP) lenses.

2. Vat dyeing involves dipping the finished lens in dye for a predetermined time. The dye penetrates only the surface, so the level of tint is independent of lens power or thickness.

3. Chemical bond tinting uses a catalyst in the soaking process to produce a stable uniform tint.

4. Printing allows an iris pattern, and a clear pupil area may also be incorporated.

Opaque tints may be produced in three ways:

1. Dot matrix printing allows some of the original iris pattern to show through.

2. Laminate construction allows the iris pattern to be protected within the lens.

3. Opaque backing is where the iris pattern and clear pupil are applied to the back of the lens, which may allow a more natural appearance.

Most translucent and opaque lenses have a clear peripheral zone so that the sclera looks natural. Opaque lenses also have a clear pupil area to avoid loss of contrast. Enhancers may incorporate a pupil area, particularly if the color is dense, but many do not, as the absence of a transition zone gives a more natural result.

For a good cosmetic result, it is desirable that the lens should not move too much, as a mobile lens may give an effect that is unsettling to an observer. Furthermore, with opaque lenses, some disruption of vision may occur if the clear pupil moves relative to that of the eye. Therefore, from an aesthetic and visual point of view, an immobile lens is ideal, and many colored lenses tend to be on the large side. However, immobility may not be a desirable characteristic from a physiologic viewpoint. It may be tricky to fit a lens that meets all of these requirements simultaneously, which may be why eye care practitioners are on the whole less enthusiastic about cosmetic lenses than are the public at large.

Tinting will affect the performance of the lens slightly in comparison with a clear lens. There may be slight effects on contrast sensitivity and on visual fields, although probably not clinically significant ones. Many patients will make the observation that flare can be a problem in low light levels when wearing 'iris' pattern lenses. Corneal edema may be slightly more likely with laminated designs, due to increased lens thickness, although most tinting processes do not affect oxygen transmission. Some tinting processes alter the surface charge of the lens surface, which could affect wettability, comfort and protein deposition, but as most colored lenses are disposable, the effects are limited.

Solutions are rarely a problem, although non-alcohol-based intensive cleaners may cause color fading. Contrary to popular belief, peroxide systems do not appear to cause fading on modern lenses, although if the lenses are worn intermittently, multipurpose solutions are a safer storage option, as they offer continuous disinfection.

UV-absorbing lenses

UV light in the bands between 315–400 nm (UVA) and 280–315 nm (UVB) has been implicated as a potential cause of cataract and macular degeneration, although the degree of risk is at present unclear. The lens absorbs most of the UV light in adults, but considerably less in children. It has been estimated that most of the UV exposure of the retina takes place before the age of 25 years, by which time the aging process of the lens provides increased protection to the retina. In young eyes, it may be that the metabolism of the retina is sufficiently robust to resist any malign effects of the exposure, whereas similar levels of radiation might cause significant damage in an older eye. Some degree of UV protection might be appropriate, then, in young patients, particularly those with light-colored irides or a lifestyle in which frequent exposure to high levels of sunlight is likely, and in post-cataract patients, who have lost the natural UV filter provided by the lens. Several lenses are available that offer enhanced UV absorption, and these may be identified from the Association of Contact Lens Manufacturers manual. It should be stressed that none of these are claimed to offer total UV protection, so in bright sunlight sunglasses are still required.

Therapeutic lenses

Most contact lenses are fitted electively, either to correct vision or for cosmetic effect, but some are fitted for therapeutic reasons. For the most part, therapeutic fitting is done in hospitals, but the practitioner may occasionally encounter such patients either in aftercare or in fitting under medical direction. The very nature of the pathologic conditions requiring therapeutic lenses means that the patient is likely to present with one or more contraindications to contact lens wear, and there is likely to be an increased risk of complications. The contraindications may be ocular, with dry eyes or epithelial compromise that would normally preclude contact lens fitting, or systemic, such as poorly controlled diabetes or arthritis. A balance must be struck between potential benefits and adverse consequences, and the patient must be kept informed of both. Lenses may need to be worn on an extended wear basis, as the normal insertion and removal procedures may disrupt an already fragile cornea. Deficient tear films may cause rapid deposition, and frequent replacement may be necessary. Various types of lens are used in therapeutic applications, both rigid and soft. The soft lenses employed have traditionally been middle-to-high water content, either custom-made or commercially available. Recently, silicone hydrogel lenses have become important, due to their combination of high oxygen permeability and resistance to deposits.

Therapeutic lenses are employed for a number of reasons:

1. correction of irregular or unusual corneal shape
2. pain relief
3. following chemical injuries
4. maintenance of a pre-corneal tear film
5. protection
6. to allow healing following trauma or surgery
7. drug delivery.

Correction of unusual or irregular corneal topography is more often associated with rigid lenses, both corneal and scleral. However, soft lenses are sometimes used successfully in early keratoconus, and in contact lens fitting following refractive surgery.

Pain relief is a relatively common reason for contact lens use. Small corneal abrasions usually heal quickly, but persistent or recurrent epithelial lesions may require a lens to protect the injury from the lid. A number of conditions may require a soft 'bandage' lens to relieve epithelial pain.

1. Recurrent erosion syndrome may follow minor trauma to the cornea, and is often associated with basement membrane dystrophy (e.g. Cogan's microcystic dystrophy, map/dot/fingerprint dystrophies). A bandage lens may prevent the lid margin from pulling on the unstable area of epithelium. This often occurs if the eyes are opened during the night or first thing in the morning, so if a lens is used, overnight wear would be most effective. Usually, lens fitting is only tried if meibomian gland dysfunction has been eliminated and ocular lubricants have failed to ameliorate the condition.
2. Epithelial dystrophies such as Reis-Buckler's, Meesman's, lattice and Fuch's dystrophies may also cause pain. In the latter stages of Fuch's dystrophy, bullous keratopathy may cause considerable pain and a bandage lens may relieve this.

3. Thygeson's superficial punctate keratopathy may be managed with a soft lens, but topical steroids are more often employed.

4. Filamentary keratitis may occur in two forms. The 'wet' variety is not accompanied by dry eye and may be seen with herpes simplex keratitis, recurrent erosion, dystonia and superior limbic keratitis. Soft lenses are often successful. However, the 'dry' form, which is accompanied by a deficient tear volume, is more often managed with rigid scleral lenses.

5. Epithelial degenerations such as Salzmann's nodular degeneration, rosacea keratopathy and atopic keratoconjunctivitis may need a soft lens for pain relief, but if conjunctival disease is also present, rigid scleral lenses may be more successful, and may improve the vision somewhat.

Following **chemical injuries**, pain relief may be provided by a soft lens, but if the limbal stem cells are destroyed, the presence of a contact lens will not prevent invasion of the cornea by epithelial cells derived from the conjunctiva. Scleral lenses may be used to maintain the fornices.

A **deficient tear layer** is usually managed with tear supplements and lubricants. The canaliculi may be blocked with punctal plugs. Hydrogel lenses tend to dry out and either tighten or fall out entirely. Silicone hydrogel lenses are more useful, having a low water content and good resistance to deposition, but often a sealed scleral lens that vaults both the cornea and limbus is a better option. It will allow the maintenance of a pre-corneal tear film, even when the corneal surface is rendered hydrophobic by dysplasia or mucus deficiency. As the lens is sealed, an RGP material is required to prevent excessive corneal edema.

Protection from the lids and the environment may be required if the lids are immobile following VIIth nerve disease, damaged by trauma or surgery, or turned in or out by chronic cicatrizing conditions such as Stevens–Johnson disease or ocular pemphigoid. Options for management include tarsorrhaphy, paralysis of the levator superioris with botulinum toxin and contact lenses, either soft lenses or scleral RGP lenses.

Following trauma or surgery, healing may be more rapid if a bandage lens protects the wound. Small aqueous leaks after trauma or trabeculectomy may be sealed, provided that the lens is large enough (up to 20 mm). Penetrating injury may be helped by the lens acting as both seal and splint. A slightly tighter fit is often used here.

Hydrogel lenses have been used to deliver 4% pilocarpine in the treatment of acute closed angle glaucoma by soaking them in the solution before insertion. Antibiotics, antivirals, epidermal growth factor and fibronectin have also been delivered in this way.

Further reading

Buckley R (2002) Therapeutic applications. In: Efron N (ed.) *Contact Lens Practice*, pp 325–331. Butterworth-Heinemann: Oxford.

Veys J, Meyler J and Davies I (2002) *Therapeutic Contact Lenses in Essential Contact Lens Practice*, pp 89–95. Butterworth-Heinemann: Oxford.

Index

A

Acanthamoeba, 154, 157–159
  clinical signs, 158
  heat disinfection, 115
  hydrogen peroxide, 117–119
  lens case, 120–121
  one-step disinfection systems, 118
  tap water, 109, 158
  treatment, 158–159
Accommodation, 71
  myopes, 5
  presbyopia, 71
Acidosis, chronic hypoxia, 86, 140
Acute closed angle glaucoma, 169
Acuvue Advance with Hydraclear
    lenses, 88–89
Acuvue lenses, 27
Acuvue Oasys with Hydraclear lenses,
    89
Adaptation, new wearers
  abnormal symptoms, 108–109
  normal symptoms, 108–109
  schedule, 107
Adnexa, general observation, 8–9
Aerosols, saline solution, 115
Aftercare, 123–133
  appointment intervals, 132–133
  background information required,
    125–127

Aftercare (*Continued*)
  compliance promotion, 129–133
  duty of care obligations, 109–110
  extended wear lenses, 95–96
  first appointment, 132
  history taking, 124–127
  lens assessment, 128
  over-refraction, 127–128
  patient information, 132
  patient reminders, 133
  purpose, 124
  symptoms/problems, 124–127
  vision assessment, 127–128
Against-the-rule astigmatism, dynamic
    stabilization, 64
Agrylamide, 27
AirOptix 89, 93
Alexidine, 120
Allergies, 3
  see also hypersensitivity reaction
Alternating squinters, monovision
    lenses, 75
Alternating vision lenses, 74
Anterior chamber activity, infections,
    155, 157, 158
Antimicrobials
  disinfection, 117–120
  dryness, 146
Appearance, perceived improvements, 6

Aspheric lenses, 59
  center-near, 78–79
Asphericity, 37–39
Assessment
  lens, aftercare, 128
  lens fit see fit assessment
  movement, 52–53
  palpebral conjunctiva, 9–11
  slit-lamp, 61, 128
  tear film, 12–15
  vision, 127–128
  see also aftercare
Astigmatic lenses, 7, 57–67
Asymptomatic infiltrates, 98, 151–152
Asymptomatic infiltrative keratitis, 98,
  152
Atopic keratoconjunctivitis, therapeutic
  lenses, 168
Axis mislocation, toric lenses, 65–66

B
Back optic zone radius (BOZR), 38
Back surface toricity, 62
Back vertex power, 39–40
Bacterial infections
  clinical signs, 156–157
  health-related factors, 155
  recurrent, 3
  risk factors, 155
  symptoms, 156
  see also specific infections/organisms
'Balanced progressive technology'
  lenses, 80
Bandage lens, 3, 167–168
Barrer ('Fatt units'), 31–32
Base-in-prism, spectacles, 5
Bausch & Lomb saline, 115
Beam movement, corneal examination,
  17–18
Bedewings (keratic precipitates), 152
Bell's phenomenon, 45
Bifocal lenses, 74, 81
Binocular contrast sensitivity, 76
Binocular inhibition, 76
Binocular summation, 76

Binocular vision decompensation,
  monovision lenses, 76
Biomicroscopes, depth perception,
  21–22
Blebs, 140
Blepharitis, 9, 143–146
  anterior, 143–144
  extended wear lenses, 91
  posterior see Meibomian gland
    dysfunction (MGD)
Blepharospasm, lens removal, 49
Blue light examination, cornea, 22–23
Blur, monovision lenses, 75–76
Boredom, non-compliance, 130
Brolene, 159
Bubbles, 13, 47, 146–147
Bulbar conjunctiva
  assessment, 11–12
  bacterial infections, 156
  hyperemia see Bulbar hyperemia
  meibomian gland dysfunction, 145
Bulbar hyperemia, 11–12, 142, 143
  infiltrative keratitis, 152
  solution intolerance reactions, 149

C
Calcium, 112
Calor, 151
Care regimes/systems, 110
  discussion, aftercare appointment,
    126–127
  dryness, 146
  non-compliance, 129–130
  see also solutions
Cataracts, UV-absorbing lenses, 166
Catarrh, 3
Center thickness, lens, 39
Center-distance (CD) lenses, 77–78
Center-near (CN) lenses, 77
  aspheric, 78–79
Chamfer, 64
'Chasing the axis', 66
Chelating agents, 112
Chemical bond tinting, 164
Chemical disinfection, 116–120

Chemical injuries, therapeutic lenses, 168

Chlorhexidine gluconate, 116–117

Chlorine-releasing agents, 117

CIBA Vision saline, 115

Citrate buffers, 114

Cleaning, 111–114
  definition, 111
  solutions see solutions

Clockwise Add, Anticlockwise Subtract (CAAS), 60

Cobalt filters, 22, 23

Collarettes, 143

Collection, 101–121
  compliance promotion, 132
  frequently asked questions, 109
  general advice, 109

'Comfort drops' (rewetting drops), 121, 146

Complete, 114

Complexion, patient, 8

Compliance
  extended wear lenses, 93
  promotion, 129–133
  repetition, 131
  see also Non-compliance

Complications, 135–159
  management strategies, 136–137

Computer numeric controlled (CNC) lathes, 78

Concretions, 11

Conjunctivitis, 10
  see also individual types

Consent forms, 108–109, 132

Consultation, initial, 1–24
  compliance promotion, 131
  goals, 2

Contact lens peripheral ulcer (CLPU), 99, 152–153

Contact lens-associated red eye (CLARE), 99, 152

Contact lens-related papillary conjunctivitis (CLPC), 11, 150
  extended wear lenses, 91, 98
  loose lenses, 52

Continuous education and training (CET), 133

Continuous professional development (CPD), 133

Contraindications, lens wear, 2–7
  therapeutic lens, 166

'Conventional lenses', 40

Copolymers (polymers), 26

Cornea
  abrasion, poor handling, 48
  abrasions
    poor handling, 47
    therapeutic lenses, 167
  blue light examination, 22–23
  chronic hypoxia, 85–86
  edema, 18
  flat, 38–39
  general examination, 15–19
  grafts, 131
  oxygen supply during sleep, 85
  sagittal height, 38–39
  specific examination, 19–22
  staining, 104–105, 145
  unusual topography, therapeutic lens use, 167
  see also entries beginning kerato-/corneal

Cornea and Contact Lens Research Unit (CCLRU) study, extended wear lenses, 93

Corneal anomaly recording, 20–22
  color, 20–21
  density, 20–21
  depth, 21–22
  location, 20
  number, 20
  size, 20

Cosmetic lenses, 162–165
  categories, 163–164
  movement, 165
  performance, 165

Cost cutting, non-compliance, 130

Crazy (fun) lenses, 163, 164

Crossed cylinder calculation, 66

Current developments, 2
Cysts, meibomian, 144–145

D

Daily disposable lens, 40
Data Protection Act, 126
Debris, tears, 13–14
Decentration, downwards (sag), 52
Depressions, beam deviation, 21–22
Diabetes, 4
Diffractive bifocal lenses, 81
Diffuse illumination, 8–9
    palpebral conjunctiva assessment,
        9–11
Dimensional stability, water content
    and, 30
Dimple veiling, 147
Direct illumination, 15, 16
Discharge, infections, 154, 156
Discomfort, 46–47, 108
    aftercare appointment, 125
    drying, 143
    excess movement, lens, 51
    toric lenses, 66–67
Disinfection, 111, 115–120
    chemical, 116–120
    heat, 115–116
Distance center multizonal lenses,
    79–80
Distance, estimation of, 20
Distance vision, center-near aspheric
    lenses, 79
Distortion, lens, 42
Dk see Oxygen permeability (Dk)
Dolor, 151
Dominant eye, monovision lenses, 75
Dot matrix printing, opaque tints, 164
Dry eye/drying, 3, 142–146
    clinical signs, 143–145
    extended wear lenses, 91
    lens surface, 125
    management, 146
    medication-induced, 4
    Rose Bengal stain, 14
    wettability, 31

Dust particles, tear film, 13
Duty of care obligations, 109–110
    out-of-hours, 96
Dye dispersion, translucent tints, 164
Dymed see Polyhexanide containing
    solutions
Dynamic stabilization (thin zone
    stabilization), 64

E

Eccentric lenticulation, 64–65
Eccentricity (shape factor), 37–38
Echelon lens, 81
Ectropion, 9
Edema
    cosmetic lenses, 165
    hypoxia, 138
    poor vision, 125
    sleep, 85
Edge damage, 125
Edge thickness, 40
EDTA (ethylene diamine tetra-acetic
    acid), 112
8 o'clock staining, 105, 148
Elevations, beam deviation, 21–22
EN ISO 11539:1999, 27–28
Endothelium, chronic hypoxia, 86, 140
Enhanced monovision, 76
Enhancers, 163, 164
Episcleritis, hyperemia, 10–11
Epithelial defects
    fluorescein examination, 22
    infections, 154
Epithelial dystrophies, therapeutic
    lenses, 167
Epithelium
    chronic hypoxia, 86, 138–140
    defects see Epithelial defects
    degeneration, therapeutic lens use,
        168
    immobile lens, 51
Erosions, 3
Ethylene diamine tetra-acetic acid
    (EDTA), 112
Ethylene glycol dimethacrylate, 27

Excess movement, lens, 51–52
Exophoria, 5
Extended wear lenses, 83–99
    adverse reactions, 96, 97–99
    aftercare, 95–96
    collection, 95–96
    demand for, 84
    diabetic patients, 4
    hazards associated with, 90–93
    history of, 84
    initial selection, 93–95
    patient suitability, 89–93
    periods of wear, 95–96
    self-assessment, 96
    solutions, 97
Extralenticular theories, presbyopia,
        71–72
Extroverts, 5
Eye
    age-related changes, 70
    anterior, sterile inflammation, 151
    approach to with lens, 46
    color, 8
        psychology, 163
    general observation, 8–9
Eye drops, intolerance reactions, 150
Eyepiece graticule, lens rotation
        measurement, 60–62

F
Fatt, Irving, 31
Fatt units (barrer), 31–32
Filamentary keratitis, therapeutic
        lenses, 168
Financial considerations, 6–7
Fingernails, lens damage, 105, 106
Fit assessment, 50–56
    aftercare appointment, 128
    good fit, 52–56
    toric lenses, 59–60
Flat toric lenses, poor vision, 66
Fluorescein, 22
    bacterial infection, 157
Fluting, extended wear lenses, 94, 95
Focimeter (lensometer), 61

Focus Aqua solution, 97
Focus Night and Day lenses, 87
    biphasic material, 87
Focus Progressive lens, 78, 80
Folds, 138
Follicles, 11–12
Food and Drug Administration (FDA)
    extended wear lenses, 84, 85
    heat disinfection approval, 115
Foreign bodies
    ferrous, 20
    infiltrative keratitis, 152
    sensation, 108
4 o'clock staining, 105, 148
Frequency 55 lens, 80
Fuch's dystrophy, 167
Fun (crazy) lenses, 163, 164

G
General health, lens wear
        contraindications/risks, 3–4
Ghost vessels, 141
    monovision lenses, 75
    toric lenses, 63, 64
Glycerylmethyl methacrylate (GMA), 27
Gram-negative bacteria
    contact lens-associated red eye, 152
    microbial keratitis, 154
Guesstimation, toric lenses, 62

H
Handling tints, 162
Hand-washing, 42, 102
Heat disinfection, 115–116
Height, presbyopia onset, 72
Hemorrhages, bacterial infections, 156
High-minus prescriptions
    center-thickness, 40
    soft *vs.* rigid gas permeable lens, 7–8
High-water lenses, center thickness, 39
Holder–Mertz criteria, extended wear,
        85, 86
Hordeolum, internal, 11, 143
Horizontal visible iris diameter (HVID),
        36, 37, 141

Hormonal changes, 4
Hot compresses, 146
Hydracare Fizzy tablets, 113
Hydraclear technology, 88–89
Hydraulic permeability, 33
Hydrocurve lenses, 27
Hydrogen peroxide, 117–119
    disadvantages, 117
    lens hydration, 118
Hydroxyethylmethacrylate (HEMA)
        lenses, 26
    edema, 67
    neovascularization, 67
Hygiene, 42, 102
    occupation, 6
    standards of, aftercare, 127
Hypercapnia, 86
Hyperemia
    bulbar conjunctiva see Bulbar
        hyperemia
    contact lens peripheral ulcer,
        152
    hypoxia, 138
    palpebral see Palpebral hyperemia
    seborrheic blepharitis, 144
Hyperopes
    lens-associated problems, 5
    presbyopia, 73
Hypersensitivity reaction, 148–150
    interpalpebral redness, 10
    secondary, 10
    staphylococcal blepharitis,
        144
Hypertension, dry eye, 4
Hypopyon, 157
Hypoxia, 137–142
    chronic, 85–86, 138–141
    clinical signs, 138–141
    corneal signs, 138
    extended wear lenses, 98
    lens material, 141–142
    lens wearing time, 141
    management, 141–142
    symptoms, 138
    toric lenses, 67

I
Immobile lens, 150
    consequences of, 51
    cosmetic, 165
    removal, 49
Indirect illumination, 15, 16
Infections, 153–159
    bacterial see Bacterial infections
    clinical signs, 156–159
    lens wear limitations, 3
    pathogenesis, 154
    symptoms, 156
    see also specific infections/organisms
Infiltrates, 19
    Acanthamoeba infection, 158
    bacterial infection, 157
    depth, 21–22
    extended wear lenses, 92
    inflammation, 151–153
    solution intolerance reactions, 149
    types, 151–153
Infiltrative keratitis, 152
    extended wear lenses, 98–99
Inflammation
    excess movement, lens, 52
    extended wear lenses, 85, 98–99
    immobile lenses, 51
    infiltrates, 19
    stages, 151
    sterile, 150–153
    see also keratitis
Informed choice, 2
Initial measurements, 36–37
'Innocent bystander' effects, 10, 19, 150
Insertion, 102–104, 107
    inspection, prior to, 103
    large surface area, 45
    lens correct way round, 43, 44, 103
    lens size, 103
    lens squashing, 46
    right lens, 103–104
    to sclera, 104
'Internet Bully', x
Introverts, 5
Ion permeability, 33

'Iris' pattern lenses, 165
Irregular astigmatism, 7
Irrigation, immobile lens removal, 49–50

K

Keeler Tearscope-Plus, 13
Keratic precipitates (bedewings), 152
Keratitis
    extended wear patients, 85
    infiltrative, 98–99, 152
    microbial *see* Microbial keratitis
    punctate, solution intolerance, 149

L

Lactation, 4
Lag, lens, 53
Laminate construction, opaque tints, 164
Lashes, general observation, 9
Lattice dystrophy, 167
Left Add, Right Subtract (LARS) rule, 60
Left-lens syndrome, 128
Lens assessment, aftercare, 128
Lens awareness
    adaptation period, 108
    drying, 143
    extended wear lenses, 97
    silicone hydrogel lenses, 97
Lens care *see* care regimes/systems
Lens case, 120–121
    age of, 127
    bacterial contamination 120
Lens design, variables in, 39–40
Lens dimensions, water loss, 55–56
Lens fitting
    spherical, 35–56
    toric, 59–60
Lens markers, 44
Lens pinching, 44, 45
Lens rotation, 59–60
    measurement, 60–62
    stabilization, 62–65
Lensometer (focimeter), 61
Lenticular theories, presbyopia, 71
Lenticulation, 64

Lesions, bacterial infection, 157
Lid(s)
    lens insertion, 46
    margin anomalies, 143–145
    position, 8
    protection, therapeutic lenses, 168
Lid scrubs, 146
Lifestyle, 6
Light green SF (lissamine green SF, wool green), 14
Limbal arcade observation, 19
Limitations, lens wear, 2–7
Lipid deposits, 128, 145, 146
Lipid solvents, 112
Lissamine green SF (wool green, light green SF), 14
Loose lenses, 51–52
Lysozyme, 114

M

Magnification
    blue light examination, 22
    initial corneal examination, 15
    low, 8–9
MAPD (myristamidopropyl dimethylamine), 119
Marginal retroillumination, microcysts, 139
Materials, 25–34
    classification, 27–28
    evaluation, 33
    hypoxia, 141–142
    see also specific materials
Mechanical abrasion, 148
Mechanical insult, 146–148
    extended wear lenses, 98
    symptoms, 146–147
Medications, dry-eye inducing, 4
Meesman's dystrophy, 167
Meibomana, 144
Meibomian cysts, 144–145
Meibomian foam, 144
Meibomian gland dysfunction (MGD), 3, 144–145

Meibomian gland dysfunction (MGD)
(Continued)
bulbar conjunctiva, 145
extended wear lenses, 91
Meibomian seborrhea, 144
Meibomitis, 144–145
management, 145
secondary seborrheic blepharitis,
145
Menopause, 4
Methacrylic acid (MA), 26–27
Methyl methacrylate (MMA), 27
Microbial keratitis, 3
extended wear lenses, 99
incidence, 153
shock tactics, non-compliant
patients, 131
smoker, 109
MicroBlock lens case, 120–121
Microcysts, 98, 137, 138–140
Microwave irradiation, 116
Mid-water lenses, center thickness, 39
Minus lenses, center thickness, 39–40
Miraflow, 112
Misinformation, non-compliance, 130
Modified monovision, 77, 80
center-distance lenses, 80
center-near lenses, 80
Monovision, 74–77
enhanced, 76
ideal patient, 75
modified see Modified monovision
partial, 76
problems, 75–76
success rate, 74–75
Motivation, for wanting lens, 5–6
Movement
assessment, 52–53
cosmetic lenses, 165
excess, 51–52
extended wear lenses, 95
Myristamidopropyl dimethylamine
(MAPD), 119
Mucin, 13
Mucin balls, 98, 147

Mucous plaques, 13
Mucous strands, tears, 13–14
Multifocal lenses, 74
pupil size, 77–78
toric, 71
Myopes
lens-associated problem, 4–5
presbyopia, 72–73

N
Naked-eye observation, 8
Near vision, center-near aspheric
lenses, 79
Neovascularization
bacterial infection, 157
chronic hypoxia, 141
extended wear lenses, 92
hydroxyethylmethacrylate lenses,
67
soft vs. rigid gas permeable lenses,
8
toric lenses, 63, 64
Neutralizing solutions, 117–118
New developments, awareness of,
133
New Fatt units, 32
Night and Day lenses, 93
Non-compliance
complications due to, 131
reasons for, 129–130, 130
shock tactics, 131
Non-invasive tear break-up time
(NIBUT), 13
'No-rub' solutions, 113–114, 119
N-vinyl pyrrolidone (NVP), 27

O
Occupation, 6
Ocular health, lens wear limitations, 3
Ocular pemphigoid, 168
Ocular surface disorders, 3
Older persons, monovision lenses, 75
Opacities, 16–17, 20
Opaque backing, 164

Opaque tints, 164
 production, 164
Opticians Act 1989 (Amendment)
        Order, 108
Opti-free, 119
Opti-free Express, 114, 119
Opti-free Supraclens solution, 113
Optim Eyes, 117
Oral contraceptives, 4
Overnight wear, 84
Over-refraction, 127–128
 center-near aspheric lenses, 79
Oxygen permeability (Dk), 31–32
 extended wear lenses, 86–87
 range codes, 28
 units, 31–32
 water content relationship, 26, 27
Oxygen transmission
 extended wear, 86–87
 lens thickness, 26
 toric lenses
Oxysept, 117–118
Oxysept 1-step system, 118

P

Pain, 125, 154
Pain, Epithelial defect, Discharge,
        Anterior chamber activity,
        Location (PEDAL) mnemonic,
        154–155
Pain relief, therapeutic lenses, 167
Palpebral conjunctiva
 assessment, 9–11
 bacterial infections, 156
 changes, extended wear lenses, 91
 grading scales, 9–10
Palpebral hyperemia, 10–11
 depth, 10–11
 solution intolerance reactions, 149
Pancreatin, 113
Papain, 113
Papillae, 12, 147–148
Papillary conjunctivitis, 147–148
 management, 148
Parallelepiped, 17, 18

Partial monovision, 76
Patient(s)
 appearance, 8
 examination, 8–23
 information/education, 108, 132
 psychological traits, 5–6
 reasons for wanting lens, 5–6
 stress, 6, 41
PEDAL (Pain, Epithelial defect,
        Discharge, Anterior chamber
        activity, Location) mnemonic,
        154–155
Perforations, 157
Perilimbal infiltrates, *Acanthamoeba*
        infection, 158
Perilimbal redness, 125
Permalens, 84
PH, effects on water content, 30
Phlycten, 10
Photophobia, 125
Pinhole, 127
Planned replacements, 40, 133, 146
Plano colored lenses, 162–163
Platinum ballasts, 5
Plus lenses, center-thickness, 40
+2.00 test, 75
Poloxamer 407, 114
Polyhexamethyl biguanide (PHMB)
        solution *see* Polyhexanide
        containing solutions
Polyhexanide containing solutions,
        114, 119
 silicone hydrogel lenses, 97
Polymegathism, 140–141
Polymeric beads, 112
Polymers, 26
Polyquad, 119
Polyquarternium 10, 114
Polyvinylpyrrolidone (PVP), 89
Poor vision *see* Vision, poor
Population, aging trends, 70
Pores, within lens, 26
Post-blink movement, extended wear
        lenses, 95
Pregnancy, 4

Presbyopia
  age of onset, 72
  causes, 71–72
  definition, 71
  ideal patient, 70–71
  soft lens for, 69–81
Printing, translucent tints, 164
Prism ballast, 5, 62–64
Prismatic correction, 5
Proclear Multifocal lenses, 80
Protein deposits, 128, 145, 146
  removal systems, 112–113, 127
    enzymes, 113
Pseudomonas aeruginosa, 154, 157
Pseudopterygium, 145
Psychological traits, patient, 5–6
Punctate keratitis, solution intolerance,
    149
Pupil diameter
  measurement, 37
  multifocal lenses, 77–78
  presbyopia onset, 72
'Pupil intelligent' design, 79
PureVision lenses, 87, 88, 93
Purilens system, 116
Purite saline, 115
Purkinje image, first, 13, 14
Push-up test, 53–55

R

Reading additions, 73
Recurrent erosion syndrome, 167
Redness, eye, 125, 143
Refraction, extended wear lenses, 98
Regard, 120
Reis–Buckler's dystrophy, 167
Reminders, aftercare appointments,
    133
Removal, 104–107
  mechanical abrasion, 148
  pinched lens, 48–49, 104–106
  soft lens, 48–50
  temporal sliding, 105, 106
ReNu MultiPlus, 97, 114
Renu with Moistureloc, 97, 114, 120

Retroillumination, 15, 16, 17
Rewetting, 121
Rewetting drops ('comfort drops'),
    121, 146
Rigid gas permeable (RGP) lenses
  alternating vision, 74
  astigmatism, 66
  complications, 136
  presbyopia, 71
  soft lens *vs.*, 7–8
  striae, 138
Ring infiltrates, 158
Rinsing, 111, 115
Risk compensation, non-compliance,
    130
Rosacea keratopathy, therapeutic
    lenses, 168
Rose bengal stain, 14
Rotation marks, toric lenses, 59, 61
'Rub-and-rinse' cleaning, 113
Rubor, 151

S

Sag (downwards decentration), 52
Saline solution
  discomfort, 46–47
  rinsing, 115
Saline tablets, 115
Salzmann's nodular degeneration, 168
SAM MF lens, 71
Scars, 19
  'bull's eye' appearance, 153
  depth, 21, 22
  extended wear lenses, 92
Sclera, lens insertion, 104
Scleritis, 11
Sclerotic scatter, 18–19
Seborrhoeic blepharitis, 144
  meibomitis, 145
Seborrhoeic dermatitis, 144
Settling period, 30, 50
  center-near aspheric lenses, 78
Shape factor (eccentricity), 37–38
Signal-to-noise ratio, multifocal lenses,
    77

Silicone hydrogel lenses, 32–33
    comfort, 88
    extended wear, 83–99
    solutions, 97
    therapeutic, 168
    toric lenses, 58–59
Silicone rubber, 33
Simultaneous vision lenses, 74
Single vision contact lenses, presbyopia, 73
Sinusitis, 3
Slab-off, 64
Sleep, corneal oxygen supply, 85
Slit-lamp assessment
    aftercare appointment, 128
    lens rotation measurement, 61
Smile stain, 91, 145
Smoking, 92, 109
'Snowflakes', 58
Sodium chlorite, 120
Sodium pyruvate, 118
Soft lens(es)
    care, 101–121
    comfort, 7
    disappearance, 50
    fitting, 35–56
    flexibility, 39–40
    fragments, 50
    handling, 41–50
    heavy, 45–46
    life span, 41
    materials see materials
    mixed up, 108
    modality, 40–41
    overuse, 129
    presbyopia, 69–81
    previous use history, 126
    replacement, 109
    right way round, 42–45
    rigid gas permeable lens vs., 7–8
    specification, 108, 126
    toric see Toric lenses
    see also entries beginning lens;
        individual lens types; specific
        indications

Solocare, 114
Solutions, 111–114
    discussion, aftercare appointment,
        126–127
    intolerance reactions, 148–150
        clinical signs, 148–149
        management, 149–150
        sterile inflammation, cornea, 150
    multipurpose, 110, 113–114, 119
    silicone hydrogel lenses, 97
    'topping up', 127, 129–130
    see also individual solutions
Spherical lenses, fitting, 35–56
Sphero-cylindrical over-refraction
    (SCO), 61, 65
Sports tints, 162
Squeeze pressure, 38, 53
Squeezy bottles, saline solution, 115
Staining
    cornea, 104–105, 145
    8 o'clock, 105, 148
    4 o'clock, 148
Staphylococcal blepharitis, 143–144
    extended wear lenses, 91
Steep lenses
    mechanical insults, 146–147
    toric, poor vision and, 66
Stereopsis, monovision lenses, 76
Sterile inflammation, cornea, 150–153
    management, 153
    triggers, 150
Sterilization, 111
Stevens–Johnson disease, 168
Stress, patient, 6, 41
Striae, 138
Stroma
    bacterial infection, 157
    chronic hypoxia, 86
Stye, 143
Subtilisin A, 113
Superior epithelial arcuate lesions
    (SEALs), 98, 147
Surface deposits, 128
Surfactants, 112
Swimming, 109

T

Tap water, 109, 130
  Acanthamoeba, 109, 158
Tear break-up time (TBUT), 13, 145
Tear film
  assessment, 12–15
  deficient, therapeutic lens use, 168
  meibomian seborrhea, 144
  solution intolerance reactions, 149
Tear lysozyme, 114
Tear prism height, 12
Tear thickness estimation, 13
Tearscopes, 13
Telangiectasia, blepharitis, 143, 144
  10-10, 118
Therapeutic lenses, 166–169
  indications, 167
  post-surgical, 169
Thermal effect, lens water content, 29
Thin zone stabilization (dynamic stabilization), 64
Thiomersal, 116–117
Thygesson's superficial punctate keratopathy, 168
Thyroid dysfunction, 4
Tight lens, 53
  toric lenses, 59
Tinted lenses, 161–169
  indications, 162
Tonicity, lens water content, 30
Toric lenses, 58
  discomfort, 66–67
  fitting, 59–60
  multifocal, 71
  problems with, 65–67
  rotation, 59–60
  stabilization, 62–65
  thickness, 66
  troubleshooting, 65–67
Total diameter, 39
Toxic reactions, 148–150
Translucent tint production, 164
Trauma
  sterile inflammation, cornea, 150
  therapeutic lenses, 169
Tris, 33
Triton Translating Bifocal, 74
Truncation, toric lenses, 64
Tumor, 151

U

Ulcers/ulceration
  Acanthamoeba infection, 158
  bacterial infection, 157
  staphylococcal blepharitis, 143
Ultrasound, 116
Ultraviolet units, 116
Ultrazyme Universal Intensive Protein Cleaner, 113
Unit dose containers, saline solution, 115
Unizyme, 113
Up-and-under approach, insertion, 46
Upper lid, lens insertion, 46
UV-absorbing lenses, 162, 165–166
Uveitis, 11

V

Vacuoles, 138–140
Vanity, patient, 5
Vat dyeing, translucent tints, 164
VDU users, enhanced monovision, 76
VIIth nerve disease, 168
N-vinyl pyrrolidone (VP), 27
Visible palpebral aperture (VPA), 37
Vision assessment, aftercare, 127–128
Vision, poor, 125
  toric lenses, 65–66
Vision, unstable, excess lens movement, 51
Visual acuity, hyperopes, 5
Visual factors, lens wear limitations, 4–5

W

Water content
  decreased, effects of, 30–32
  Dk relationship, 26, 27
  factors influencing, 29–33

Watermelon seed principle, 64
Wear patterns, 107, 126
    adaptation schedule, new wearers,
        107
    extended see Extended wear lenses
Weekly disposable lenses, 85
Wettability, 30–31
White light investigation, aftercare
        appointment, 128
Wool green (lissamine green SF, light
        green SF), 14

Worst case scenario, complications,
        137
Written information, 108, 132

Y
Yellow filters, 22

Z
Zipper effect, 62

183